1

WHY PERSONALIZED MEDICINE?

EARLY ONE MORNING Jonathan, twelve years old, wakes up and finds that his stomach hurts—hurts badly. But he has no temperature and is not nauseous; he's just in a lot of pain. His mother, Marianne, is not alarmed at first, only irritated that she can't go to work. She lets Jonathan stay home from school, assuming that all will be well come evening. But the pain persists. By evening, she thinks perhaps seeing the doctor is a good idea; by early morning, after a night of sitting by Jonathan's bed, listening to him moan, going to emergency has become a necessity. After an interminable wait in the emergency room, Jonathan is finally examined by a doctor. The doctor gently prods and probes Jonathan's abdomen and then starts to look worried. He orders a CT scan. Marianne, who is now very apprehensive, asks, "What's wrong?" The doctor is noncommittal: "Let's wait for the scan."

But bad news follows. There is a mass in Jonathan's stomach, the size of a golf ball. At this point, Marianne is having trouble holding herself together, and she calls her husband, Bill, who immediately races to the hospital. He feels sick at heart—the dreaded "cancer" word has not been spoken yet, but it is in the air.

The news gets worse. Jonathan is admitted to hospital, a biopsy is performed, cancer is diagnosed, and surgery followed by chemotherapy is advised. Jonathan's life is at stake. The surgery is as successful as it can be, but it is very rare that a surgeon can remove all of this type of cancer. Hence the chemotherapy, to try to kill any remaining cancer cells.

Jonathan reacts well to the first dose of chemotherapy. He feels tired but does not get sick. Bill and Marianne allow themselves to dream: maybe Jonathan will get through this, and life will become a little more normal again. But following the second dose, Jonathan becomes short of breath after walking only a few steps. Back to the emergency: this time, the doctor calls a cardiologist, who tests Jonathan's heart using an echocardiograph. The cardiologist returns, grim faced. "Your son has heart failure," he informs Marianne and Bill. It turns out that Jonathan is highly sensitive to one of the drugs in the chemotherapy used to treat him. The drug, doxorubicin, causes heart problems in some patients,[1] but the doctors have no way of knowing which patients are going to be affected.

In the space of a month, Jonathan has been transformed from a normal twelve-year-old to an invalid undergoing cancer treatment who also needs a heart transplant. How did this happen? The presence of a tumor the size of a golf ball indicated a cancer that had been growing for at least three years. Why couldn't it have been detected long before, when it would have been much easier to treat?

And why was Jonathan treated with a drug that caused his heart to fail?

These "adverse drug reactions" are common: every year more than 2 million North Americans are hospitalized because of adverse reactions to prescription drugs.[2] The reason why drugs work in some people and cause bad reactions in others can usually be traced back to differences in genetic makeup. Medicines that work for most people may not work for you. They may, indeed, harm you. So we need two things: first, we need ways of predicting and detecting disease well before it becomes life threatening; and second, we need medicines that work for you and your unique body.

Medicine has been trying to do these two things for millennia. While enormous progress has been made, it is still not good enough. And so it is that we are nearing the biggest revolution of our time—perhaps of all time.

This revolution has many names and guises. It is sometimes called personalized medicine, sometimes precision medicine, sometimes stratified medicine. It is a cousin of "evidence-based" medicine, a relatively new concept in medical practice. (Whoever came up with that name was clearly trying to make a point.) Whatever the name, what we will call personalized medicine—medicine based on the unique molecular makeup of our individual selves and a molecular-level understanding of whatever disorder we may have—is on our doorsteps. It promises to satisfy our need to know what is wrong with us and provide ways to treat our ailments that our species has been seeking since the beginning of recorded time. It will also mean that once and for all, we will leave behind the natural evolutionary forces that our ancestors endured and embark on a self-directed future.

We tend to view medical progress as some sort of continuum, along which we develop better drugs to fight whatever diseases are prevalent, better machines to image our insides and detect problems, better devices to use when joints wear out or eyes fail, better ways to treat pain or depression or loneliness; and we might be inclined to believe that the future holds more of the same. But it is not going to happen that way.

Medical progress to this point has been mainly based on advances that benefit the population as a whole rather than you as an individual. Two hundred years ago, the average life span in England was only about forty years, largely because two-thirds of all children died before age four.[3] Public-health initiatives leading to adequate diet and clean water have had a huge impact, and these, combined with other population-wide advances such as vaccination, sterile procedures during childbirth and surgery, and antibiotics to treat bacterial diseases mean that the average life span today is about eighty years or more. But population-based approaches to maintain human health and life have begun to fail.

The most obvious way current medicine has begun to fail is in the development of drugs. When Paul Ehrlich discovered arsphenamine, a drug to treat syphilis, in 1909 and introduced the concept of the "magic bullet" to cure our illnesses, and when Alexander Fleming followed up with the discovery of penicillin in 1928 to cure a wide spectrum of infectious diseases, we became seduced by the notion that other compounds could be found that would have similar magical effects on other diseases, ranging from cancer to the common cold. An enormous industry, the pharmaceutical industry, has sprung up as a result, and there are now more than a thousand commonly prescribed drugs to treat almost every disease you can name. The average family doctor in North America writes more than 20,000 prescriptions for these drugs every year. This practice has led to alarming levels of medication, with approximately 20 percent of North Americans over the age of sixty-five taking ten or more drugs every day. More than 50 percent of Americans take at least one prescription drug each day.[4] As a direct result, the fourth highest cause of death in North America is a bad reaction to a drug or drug regimen, resulting in more than 100,000 deaths per year.[5] Furthermore, it has been estimated that up to 90 percent of adverse drug reactions are not reported,[6] so the dangers associated with taking prescription drugs are likely much higher.

In addition to the potential for causing a bad reaction, many of these drugs simply do not work for the individual who takes them. The numbers are appalling. Approximately 75 percent of drugs for cancer treatment do not help the patient they are prescribed for. More than 70 percent of the drugs for Alzheimer's do not work on the patient they are prescribed for. Nearly 60 percent of drugs for incontinence are of little use to the patient they are prescribed for. Fifty percent of drugs for osteoporosis do not lead to stronger bones in the patient they are prescribed for. Rheumatoid arthritis, migraine, cardiac arrhythmia, asthma—more than 40 percent of the drugs used to treat these conditions do not work on the patient they are prescribed for. In general, less than 50 percent of prescribed drugs actually help the patient they are prescribed for.[7]

There are problems even with drugs that are hugely successful. Statins, "blockbuster" drugs used to treat high levels of blood cholesterol, have been found to reduce the risk of a heart attack by 54 percent and the risk of a stroke by 48 percent.[8] They have been instrumental in reducing deaths due to cardiovascular disease to the point where it is now no longer the leading cause of death in the Western world. On average, for most people, statins work very well.

However, the problem with statins and other blockbuster drugs is that many people aren't average. Some people metabolize statins too quickly: their bodies break down the medication before it gets a chance to work, and their cholesterol levels stay high, so they are still at increased risk of a heart attack or stroke. Others metabolize the drug too slowly, and it lingers in their systems, lowering cholesterol levels but also causing all sorts of uncomfortable, often painful, side effects. It has been estimated that 17 percent of statin users suffer from muscle pain and nausea.[9] The really unlucky ones can have serious reaction to the drug, statin-induced rhabdomyolysis,[10] a debilitating form of muscle damage, which can result in kidney failure.

Adverse drug reactions occur because most common drugs go everywhere in your body. Only a small proportion, usually far less than 1 percent, ends up at a disease site where it can have a beneficial effect. The other 99 percent can cause problems in previously healthy tissues. Doxorubicin, a commonly prescribed anticancer drug, is very effective for killing rapidly dividing cells such as cancer cells, but because it goes everywhere, it also kills rapidly dividing cells in your bone marrow, causing your immune system to be compromised; in your stomach lining, causing you to throw up; and in your hair cells, causing your hair to fall out. All this is in addition to the severely toxic effects it can have on your heart.

There are still more problems. One of the first major successes of cancer chemotherapy was in treating childhood leukemia. In 1950, a diagnosis of leukemia in childhood was an almost certain death sentence, with more than 90 percent of children dying within a year.[11] Now more than 90 percent of children who are diagnosed with acute lymphoblastic leukemia, the most common type of childhood cancer, are cured, judging by the number of patients who remain cancer free for five years after treatment. But these survivors often do not lead normal lives. More than 30 percent of children treated with the most effective drug cocktail go stone deaf, permanently.[12] Other "side effects" include infertility, retardation—the list goes on and on. The costs to the child are immeasurable, emotionally damaging, and career limiting. The costs to society are daunting: often more than $20,000 per child per year until adulthood to provide special resources.

This example is not an isolated one. The common chemotherapy protocol for treatment of solid cancers in children calls for doxorubicin. It is not unusual for a child being treated for such cancers to go into heart failure as a result of chemotherapy, which sometimes makes a heart transplant necessary. More often, the effects of a weakened heart persist through the survivor's lifetime.

Drugs to treat many conditions are hit or miss: a family practice physician, on being asked how he selects the best drug for patients suffering from depression, answered, "Well, I have a dartboard hanging behind my door. It depends what number I hit." There is no way for him to know in advance which drug will work best for which patient and which patient will suffer a nasty side effect. And so the patient and the doctor embark on a risky trial-and-error journey to find the best, most effective drug for him or her.

The problems arising from the variable efficacy of drugs and their toxic side effects on healthy tissues have made the development of new drugs an almost impossible task: getting a drug approved now costs more than $1 billion and may take more than fifteen years.[13] Even then, some adverse reaction that occurs in a small subset of people may cause the drug to be withdrawn from the market.

All these problems spring from a one-size-fits-all approach to medicine. This approach doesn't necessarily work, because what you have always thought about yourself is actually true: you really are different from everybody else. And you need to be treated appropriately. The medicine of the future is going to be much more personalized—designed specifically for you and the body you inhabit.

Doctors are often upset by the term personalized medicine. "We have always practiced personalized medicine!" they proclaim, meaning that they listen to and consult with their patients and diagnose and advise on an individual basis. And so they do. But how much do they actually know about you? Your doctor sees the macroscopic version of you and, on the basis of a physical examination and your symptoms, can often diagnose what is wrong quite efficiently. But your doctor does not know much about the microscopic version of you, where disease and your responses to treatment are first manifested. Your doctor does not know details of your genetic code and therefore cannot know how you will respond to a drug he or she may prescribe. Your doctor does not know the composition of molecules in your blood, which contain a huge amount of diagnostic information regarding diseases that you may have or be trending towards, whether the drugs you are taking are working to cure whatever disorder you are suffering from, or whether your diet is appropriate. Your doctor does not know the types and amounts of micro-organisms that are living in you and on you, which influence how well your immune system is working and play important roles in inflammatory diseases. In short, your doctor does not have access to a lot of important molecular-level information about you to guide many of his or her decisions. This can lead to wrong or delayed diagnoses and inappropriate therapeutic interventions.

The medicine of the future will be more personalized—and much more effective—because detailed molecular-level information about you and whatever disorder you may have is increasingly available. The lead example is your genome— your DNA (deoxyribonucleic acid), which codes for every physical feature you have and which makes you the individual you are, with all your strengths and weaknesses. Soon it will be normal for you to have your genome sequenced, to decipher the molecular code contained in the long strings of DNA found in your cells, and have this information stored as part of your medical record. The sequence of your genome contains detailed and accurate information on your risk for diseases ranging from heart disease to diabetes, to depression and dementia, as well as information as to which drugs might work best for you and which might produce harmful side effects.

However, the sequence of your genome does not give complete information about you. With the exception of genetic diseases such as cancer and inherited conditions, genomic sequences are not that useful for diagnosing disorders you actually have—and that's where proteomics, the next level of molecular analysis, kicks in. Your genome codes for the proteins that make you the animal that you are; and all the proteins in your body constitute what's called your proteome. We're getting pretty good at measuring your proteome—which is important, because an analysis of, say, 1,000 proteins in your blood or other bodily fluid will potentially provide an accurate diagnosis of any disease you actually have or are trending towards. Such analyses will also be able to tell you whether the therapy you're undergoing or the lifestyle change you're making is helping you to regain your health.

And so it goes on: an avalanche of molecular-level analyses of the bits and pieces that make up you is coming online. Within the next five years, increasingly comprehensive molecular tests will be available that will tell you, with ever-improving accuracy, what is wrong with you when you don't feel well or are in pain or are depressed or feel weak. A hypochondriac's heaven—or hell, depending on your point of view.

For those who want a monitored life, it is going to be heaven. Wristbands, implants, or a high-tech Band-Aid will be able to give you minute-by-minute reports of your physical status, and you'll be able to download these to your computer to see day-to-day and longer trend lines. This degree of monitoring means a big change in preventive health care, or maintaining wellness. Soon you will have data that tells you whether that probiotic stuff you hate is working as advertised, whether those three drinks a day you crave are doing any harm—or good—or whether that gym membership is worth it. Elite athletes will be early adopters: for those always training at a level just shy of doing themselves injury, a voice in their ear saying their left calf muscle is going to tear in five minutes if they don't slow down or that their energy reserves are good for another thirty minutes at that pace, but no longer, would be most welcome.

This future is not far away. Many of the technologies that will allow truly personalized medicine are either in place or close to it. You have probably heard about many of them—nearly every day we hear of some advance in determining the molecular basis of one cancer or another or the development of drugs that can cure patients with genetic diseases such as cystic fibrosis. These announcements are usually accompanied by a solemn pronouncement that "these findings could lead to new medicines to treat disease within five years" or some variant thereof, and then you never hear about it again.

We have become inured to such announcements, thinking that they will never apply to us. But they will—and soon.

2

FROM MAGICAL THINKING TO PERSONALIZED MEDICINE

WHEN PEOPLE DON'T understand things that are clearly important, they often resort to magical thinking, otherwise known as making stuff up. Inventing deities to explain the world around us was a favorite occupation of our ancestors. Mayans would sacrifice virgins at dawn as the sun rose over the Atlantic, blood-red from its battles in the underworld of night, to celebrate yet another victory of the sun god. For the Greeks, thunder and lightning expressed the displeasure of Zeus, the god of the sky. In Chinese mythology, clouds were the breath of the dragon kings. The Indian god Indra brought on the monsoon rains by defeating Vritra, the Demon of Drought, who held the "cloud-cattle" captive in his mountain fortress. Creation was explained by the Apache gods Tepeu and Gucumatz, who sat together and thought, and whatever they thought came into being. They thought "Earth!"—and there it was. And on it goes, every civilization inventing fascinating myths to explain everything from the origins of the universe to the stars in the sky and what happens after death.

Disease and pain are particularly effective for inducing magical thinking. In medieval Europe, Christians thought the bubonic plague to be a punishment for man's wicked ways. Self-flagellation, to atone for one's sins, was therefore seen as a logical means to avoid the Black Death. In fifteenth-century Japan, disease was believed to be caused by horrible little creatures living inside you. Dizziness and hot flashes were caused, for example, by an animal living in your spleen called Hizonomushi, which could cause problems by grabbing your muscles with its long arms and claws. Luckily, Hizonomushi could be tamed if you ate rhubarb. To ancient Egyptians, illnesses were caused by the presence of evil spirits. Cleansing the body by incantations, prayers to Sekhmet, the goddess of healing, and the injection of nasty-tasting medicines into various bodily orifices to drive the evil spirits out, were prescribed treatments.

We still indulge in remarkable levels of magical thinking when our health is threatened. Folk remedies for everything from treatment of the common cold to cancer are followed with zeal. Apple cider vinegar for treatment of allergies, acid reflux, gout, arthritis, headaches, yeast infections, psoriasis, you name it. Banana peels for warts, beets for constipation, Epsom salts for nail fungus—there are loyal proselytizers for all these "cures." Herbal remedies are used to treat depression, heart disease, insomnia, hypertension, and weight gain. Twenty thousand herbal medicines are available in the United States, and these are used by more than 80 million people. However, there is very limited evidence that even the ten most commonly used remedies are at all effective, and harmful side effects can be significant.[1] There are even believers in the benefits of homeopathic medicine, who strain credulity when they tell us that giving less of a therapeutic is somehow supposed to result in improved therapy.

This level of magical thinking is inconceivable in almost all other areas of our lives. You certainly wouldn't accept that a plane crash was caused by bad karma or that your boat sank because you offended the god of the sea. But when it comes to our health, we give our imagination full rein. There is good reason for this, of course: When there are no explanations or cures for things that are sometimes terribly wrong, what else can we do? We consult the high priests of medicine about our ailments; they consider, discuss, and prescribe; sometimes things work and sometimes they don't. We feel ourselves to be helpless cogs in a giant medical processing plant that we do not understand and are powerless to resist, and magical thinking is our only resort.

Personalized medicine, which we will also call molecular medicine, is the antithesis of magical thinking. It is driven by the conviction that every ailment you have has a cause at the molecular level and that once you understand the cause of your disorder, an appropriate molecular-level treatment can be devised that will work for you. It is also driven by the conviction that signals of disease are apparent well before the disease appears (at which point it may be too late). We simply need to recognize what those signals are.

The road from magical thinking to personalized medicine has been blazed by the development and application of modern science, an odyssey that began less than 500 years ago.

The story begins with Galileo Galilei, born in Pisa, Italy, in 1564. He is generally accepted to be the father of modern science. He was the first scientist to note that the universe is constantly changing, the first to observe that moons could orbit around planets, and the most effective in championing the view that the Earth could be orbiting the sun. Because of his inability to accept the magical thinking that put the Earth at the center of the universe, he was found "vehemently suspect of heresy" by the Roman Inquisition and put under house arrest by the Catholic Church for the last nine years of his life. Galileo was also the first to postulate in clear terms that mathematics is key to understanding the universe. Galileo stated that "the universe...cannot be understood unless one first learns to comprehend the language and interpret the characters in which it is written. It is written in the language of mathematics...without which it is humanly impossible to understand a single word of it; without which, one is wandering around in a dark labyrinth." This statement is fundamental to all progress that has been made since Galileo's death, in 1642, in determining what we are made of and how it works. There is little doubt that if there is a God, the language that He/She/It speaks is mathematics. Anyone who has experienced the eerie, unearthly, completely alien precision with which mathematics can be used to describe the universe from the beginning of time to the end of time, from the very smallest particle to the very largest galaxy, has a sense of this.

Isaac Newton was born in a small village near Cambridge, England, in the year in which Galileo died. He lived in Cambridge and London and during his lifetime, drove a dagger into the heart of magical thinking. He did it by taking Galileo's approach to heart, developing sophisticated mathematics that allowed him to marry mathematics with natural philosophy and thereby inventing modern physics. He invented classical mechanics and calculus to explain the motion of suns and planets and devised a theory of optics to explain how light works. Before Newton, everything was magic; but by using his classical mechanics, people came to understand that eclipses occurred because the moon gets between the Earth and the sun, that the sea rises and falls because of the gravitational pull of the moon and the sun, and that seasons happen because of the Earth's axial tilt. Furthermore, he proved that if you get accurate data, construct the right model, and do the mathematics correctly, you can predict when high tides will happen, when eclipses will occur, when comets will blaze across the sky, and when they will return. Magic reigned no more.

How does this apply to you? The classical mechanics Newton invented to understand the movement of planets, as well as apples falling from trees, also applies to the world of the very small, down to distances as little as one billionth of a meter (a nanometer), at which point quantum mechanics takes over. Since the molecules and cells in your body are bigger than a nanometer, classical mechanics can be used to describe and predict the ways the molecules in your body move and interact, which is basic to the construction and interpretation of you at the molecular level. But Newton's work is far more pro-found than that. By the time he died in 1727, we had the sure knowledge that we can understand natural phenomena by first measuring them very accurately, then building a theoretical, mathematical model that fits with these observations, and finally by conducting experiments to test other predictions of the theory to see if it is generally true. This approach is the most fertile discovery process the world has ever known.

Antonie van Leeuwenhoek was a contemporary of Newton's, although they never met. He was born in Holland in 1632 and was the first person to show that while you may think of your-self as a continuous whole, there are many little bits of you. Leeuwenhoek made powerful microscopes that could magnify by as much as 500 times, allowing him to see individual cells. In a series of reports to the Royal Society of London, he described the microscopic world for the first time, including bacterial cells he found in any body of water he looked at, the bacteria he found in his mouth and feces, blood cells he found in blood vessels, sperm cells he found in "recent ejaculate from a healthy man," the organized arrays of cells he found in muscle, and so on. Leeuwenhoek's discoveries showed that to understand you, we first need to understand what goes on in the cells you're composed of.

What *does* go on in the cells that you're made of? The initial steps to address this question were taken by a French Anthony, namely Antoine Lavoisier, who was born in 1743 in Paris, where he remained all his life. Lavoisier was interested in how things burned and why air is necessary for things to burn. Through a careful series of experiments that signified the start of modern chemistry, he determined that when things burn, a component of air is consumed to produce carbon dioxide. The component that is consumed is now known as oxygen, and as a result, the process of burning is often referred to as oxidation. Lavoisier then showed in a remarkably intuitive experiment that when an animal breathes, it produces exactly the same amount of heat per amount of oxygen consumed and amount of carbon dioxide produced as any other combustion process.

Thus was born the idea that a constant process of slow burning, or oxidation, takes place in our bodies, where the food that we eat is the fuel that we burn. This discovery explained why our bodies are warm and led to subsequent discoveries of how oxidation is used to provide power for movement, thought, and sight—in short, for all bodily functions. Lavoisier's contribution to understanding ourselves was profound; however, he had the misfortune to be a wealthy and influential man in Paris at the time of the French Revolution. He was guillotined in 1794 after being convicted of corruption on trumped-up charges. He was pardoned a year later, but by then it was a little too late.

Lavoisier was followed by another giant in the evolution of chemistry: John Dalton, who invented the atomic theory and the idea that elements combine to form molecules consisting of fixed ratios of these elements to make liquids, such as water, and gases, such as carbon dioxide. Dalton was born in 1766 in England and spent most of his life in Manchester, dying there in 1844, just after a statue was erected in his honor in the town square. The combined work of Lavoisier and Dalton gave rise to modern chemistry, including biochemistry, which describes the way that biological molecules, such as proteins coded for by your DNA, do their work inside cells.

Charles Darwin was also vitally important in the quest to understand what you're made of. He was born in 1809 and managed in his lifetime to establish the fundamental reality that humans and all other life forms are related to each other by a vicious selection process known as evolution, in which only those species most adapted to their environment survive. The concept of survival of the fittest permeates to the very heart of you: each molecule in your body has evolved through millennia to function as well as possible to ensure that species that preceded you could survive. Mechanisms that were honed over 4,000 million years of evolution in species ranging from bacteria, sponges, worms, fish, and vertebrates have been adapted in your body in more ways than you can imagine. For example, every cell in your body contains little fuel cells called mitochondria. Mitochondria perform the oxidation process first noted by Lavoisier and produce molecules called adenosine triphosphate (ATP) by burning molecules derived from the food you eat. The ATP, in turn, provides power for your body to function. Mitochondria are direct descendants of an early bacterium that evolved to live in a symbiotic manner in cells that were precursors of the cells making up your body. Without mitochondria, we could not exist.

Your ability to see depends on the evolution of proteins that can detect light. Vision evolved during a relatively short period of evolutionary time (400,000 years) from primordial light-sensing proteins that enabled unicellular organisms to orient towards the sun. When versions of these proteins were somehow incorporated into animals to enable them to see, organisms that couldn't see became lunch for animals that could.

Charles Darwin could have used some personalized medicine. The list of ailments that tortured him throughout his life are legion and include "malaise, vertigo, dizziness, muscle spasms and tremors, vomiting, cramps and colics, bloating and nocturnal intestinal gas, headaches, alterations of vision, severe tiredness, nervous exhaustion, dyspnea, skin problems such as blisters all over the scalp and eczema, crying, anxiety, sensation of impending death and loss of consciousness, fainting, tachycardia, insomnia, tinnitus, and depression."[2] There are tales that he suffered from uncontrollable flatulence that caused him to retire to his study for at least an hour after dinner. Nonetheless, he was one of the giants, up there with Newton and Galileo, in the battle against magical thinking. His theory of evolution allowed us to discover ourselves by analyzing simpler organisms such as yeast, flies, and mice to see what makes them—and you—tick. This work has led to the discovery of DNA as the molecular mechanism whereby biological information can be passed on from generation to generation, the discovery and characterization of early versions of the cells and molecules that you are made of, and the discovery and development of all the ways we have to treat disease.

In parallel with the exploits of Leeuwenhoek, Lavoisier, Dalton, and Darwin in understanding the biological world, progress was also being made in understanding the physical world, again based on the example Newton set. An important example is electricity, which is not just vital to our civilization but also vital to every device we use to characterize you and to interpret the vast amounts of information that result. Two pioneering scientists who enabled us to use electricity were Michael Faraday and James Maxwell. Faraday discovered that electric currents were associated with magnetic fields. He made the first electrical motor when he showed that a changing electrical field could exert a force on a magnet in that field, and he hypothesized that magnets (and wires carrying electrical currents) had invisible fields associated with them, which he called lines of force.

James Maxwell, who was born in Edinburgh in 1831, was a direct intellectual descendant of Newton in that besides trying to understand natural phenomena, he was also one of the best mathematicians of his time. He invented the new mathematics required to understand the relationship between magnetism and electricity. He showed that Faraday's lines of force had a tangible reality that could be modeled theoretically. He came up with Maxwell's laws, which solved electromagnetic behavior for all time, and allowed us to generate and transmit electricity and to use it in all the electronic gadgets we are so familiar with today. His work also led to wireless transmission of information, ranging from radio to television, to the wireless connection your cell phone uses. Maxwell was only forty-eight when he died, but like Newton, he changed the world, moving electricity from the curiosity of static electricity or the drama of lightning into something we could understand, harness, and use. Aside from enabling the machines we use to characterize all the molecules that make you up, Maxwell's equations also apply to the electrical currents that are used by the nerves in your body to make your hands move on demand or your heart beat or your brain think.

There is another important stream of intellectual endeavor that has led to a greater understanding of our molecular selves:

technology, or the application of science to produce things of practical use. Galileo and Newton developed technology by grinding lenses and building telescopes so they could examine the heavens in detail and see whether their theories were compatible with observation. The tradition of building ever more sophisticated instruments to investigate natural phenomena has become deeply ingrained in science, particularly physics, and has led to every single one of the machines we use today. Technology received a decided boost when Maxwell found out how we could tame electricity and has since gone on to define our civilization.

But how does the development of technology apply to personalized medicine? The answer lies in the computers we use to collect and decipher the molecular information describing you, the machines we use to visualize what is going on inside you, and the ways in which we can transmit information about you.

Without computers, the notion of molecular medicine could not exist. Computers are used every step of the way, from controlling the instrumentation that we use to decipher your DNA, for example, to storing the immense amounts of data that we get from molecular-level analyses of DNA, proteins, and other biological molecules, to analyzing all this data so that we can use it to benefit you. But we haven't always had computers. How did they come to be? The imaginings of Charles Babbage and the brilliance of Alan Turing played a large part. Babbage was born in London in 1791 and is considered the "father of the computer," although he only ever had one working model, and it was very limited. Babbage had a great many interests, being a mathematician, philosopher, astronomer, economist, inventor, theologian, cryptographer, and engineer. He also wrote a variety of articles for popular consumption on "public nuisances" such as the abominable nature of street music to the role of drunkenness in women and boys as the cause of broken windows. Obviously, a lot of things, including many people, bothered Babbage.

One thing that particularly bothered Babbage was that mathematical tables necessary for navigation, the forecasting of tides, or computation were full of errors, as the numbers were derived by "computers"—which, at that time, were human beings. Babbage thought that one way to eliminate these mistakes would be to have the tables generated by machines designed for the task, and he set about designing such an instrument, drawing on his considerable engineering talents. The result was the "difference machine"—a mechanical computer having 15,000 parts and weighing 10 tons. The difference machine was, in fact, never built in Babbage's lifetime, but it was completed some 150 years later by following Babbage's original plans—and it worked.

Alan Turing, who was born in 1912 in London, had an enormous influence on the design of computers. In 1935, he published a scientific paper that demonstrated that any computation that can be reduced to a set of instructions can be done by a computer, subsequently called a Turing machine. He also played a major role in winning the Second World War by designing the early mechanical computers that broke the German cryptography codes. This allowed the British to read the transmissions of the German army, navy, and air force. Alan Turing and other cryptographers worked at Bletchley Park, north of London. As Winston Churchill put it, Bletchley Park was "the goose that laid the golden egg—and never cackled."

Turing did not receive much thanks for his amazing contributions. He was homosexual, which led to his arrest in 1952 on charges of gross indecency. His security privileges were revokcd, and criminal charges were brought against him. He was given a choice of prison or chemical castration, and he chose castration. He committed suicide in 1954. The British Government gave an official apology to Alan Turing in 2009, but as with Antoine Lavoisier, it was a little too late.

The Turing machine envisioned and built by Alan Turing anticipated and led to all the computers we use today. The ones we use now, however, are a great deal more powerful, much more compact, much easier to make, much cheaper, and much more personal. How did this happen? It is here that we get into microtechnology and nanotechnology, and we can start to see how the grand design of nature's technology (the molecules and nanomachines that make up you)—which was arrived at by evolutionary forces—and the technology that arises from the findings of Newton, Maxwell, and Darwin are converging. Both the natural and the human-made technologies are aimed at perfecting machinery that functions in the world of the very small.

It is important to start to think in terms of the world of the very small. It is crucial to understanding how technology has evolved to produce all the devices we see around us, particularly the devices we use to store and process data about you. It is also vital to understanding yourself, as you consist of an enormous number of exquisitely designed nanomachines. The computers we design are decreasing in size as we cram more and more functions into smaller and smaller spaces. This trend was predicted by Richard Feynman in 1959 when he gave a lecture that signaled the start of the information age. The lecture was entitled "There's Plenty of Room at the Bottom," a brilliant title for a deeply profound insight into nature. Richard Feynman was one of the most influential thinkers of the twentieth century. He played a key role in the Manhattan Project, which produced the atomic bomb, and he won a Nobel Prize in 1965 for his work on quantum theory. Fellow physicists held Feynman in awe because of his remarkable computational abilities and his unique ways of solving problems. When asked how Feynman solved problems, one colleague commented, "Well, he thinks really, really hard and then tells you the answer." He was an unusual person—his favorite hobbies were cracking safes and playing bongo drums, and he found the atmosphere of a local strip bar to be most beneficial for productive thought.

Feynman certainly pointed out that very large amounts of information could be stored and analyzed in very small devices. Through a simple series of calculations, he demonstrated that without breaking any of the laws of nature, it should be possible to store the entire contents of the Library of Congress, together with addresses indicating where that information is stored, in a particle smaller than a speck of dust. The computers and smartphones we use now illustrate how far we have come in realizing this goal: compared with early computers such as Colossus—which was built in 1944 and was the size of an average office—today's laptop is at least a billion times more powerful. And we still have a long way to go before we hit the limits that Feynman identified.

The key to making computers smaller was the invention of the transistor. Until 1950, the only way we could control electrical currents to make devices such as radios or TVs was by using glass vacuum tubes that housed electrical circuits that regulated the flow of electricity through the tube. These tubes were large, the size of a shot glass or bigger, and lots of them were required—which resulted in computing machines the size of Colossus, with enormous energy demands. William Shockley, in partnership with John Bardeen and Walter Brattain, invented the transistor in 1947, which changed everything. Shockley also demonstrated that brilliant people are not necessarily that enlightened: he had distinctly bigoted views. He believed, for example, that the human race was being degraded because poorer people with limited intellectual capabilities were having too many children. The transistor, however, was an enormous contribution. Transistors can be configured to be in an "on" state (current can flow through) or an "off" state (no current flows through), and are therefore ideally suited to storing information in the binary code (zeros or ones) that all computers use today. In addition, the main component used in transistors is silicon, also known as sand, so costs can be low. Finally, the circuits that make up transistors can be miniaturized so that massive amounts of processing power and information can be stored in very little space.

The first transistor was very large by current standards— about the size of a small postage stamp. Today, a single transistor can be more than a thousand times smaller. By putting transistors together in appropriate ways, the functions of complete circuits can be achieved, and by putting a lot of these circuits together as one physical entity, integrated circuits that perform specific functions (such as detection of radio waves, amplification, data storage, and so on) can be made. Interestingly, the length scale of the circuitry in today's integrated circuits is approaching the length scale of the machinery in your body's cells, which operates on the nanometer scale. In 1990, the smallest circuit components had dimensions of 500 nanometers, which were reduced to 45 nanometers by 2010 and are now approaching 10 nanometers. We are nowhere near being able to match the complexity of biological nanotechnology, which has been honed by eons of evolution, but we are getting closer.

So Newton's work led to Maxwell's insights, Shockley's transistor, and Feynman's predictions, which in turn led to Bill

Gates, Steve Jobs, and the computers, smartphones, and other devices we know and love. Thanks to this progression, we now have ways of storing and analyzing enormous amounts of information. And Lavoisier, Dalton, and Darwin laid the groundwork for modern biochemistry, and thus a molecular-level understanding of living organisms began to evolve.

Still, how is it that we have found ways of detecting, characterizing, and measuring all the molecules that make you up? It's through application of all the technology we've developed to make everything from computers to smartphones, to the cars we drive, to the movies we watch. This technology is now sufficiently advanced that it can be used to decipher you at the molecular level.

The application of technology to biology started slowly but is now ramping up to warp speed. Early examples were the microscopes invented by Leeuwenhoek, but it wasn't until the discovery of X-rays by Wilhelm Röntgen in 1895 that things really took off. The discovery of X-rays led to many things, two of which are vital to personalized medicine. First, X-rays provided a way to look inside you—as was noted by Röntgen. The first X-ray picture ever taken was one by Röntgen of his wife's hand. On seeing the skeletal structure, she exclaimed, "I have seen my death!" Today, you take the ability to image things inside your body for granted, but up until 1900, it was impossible. X-ray machines have been used for all sorts of things, including by shoe stores to see how well your shoes fit—definitely not the most inspired of applications. Now we have all sorts of ways to look inside ourselves, including sophisticated X-ray machines called computed tomography (CT) scanners, which give remarkable three-dimensional visualizations of bones, tissues, and tumors in your body; magnetic resonance imaging (MRI) machines, which give images with excellent resolution for soft tissues such as the brain; and ultrasound imaging, which allows you to look at your baby before it is born.

The second way that X-rays are vital to personalized medicine is that they can be used to determine the structure of the molecules you are made of. Linus Pauling, one of only four people who have won two Nobel prizes, was the first to develop this application. Pauling became a professor at the California Institute of Technology in 1927 and was a polymath who excelled at everything he did, although he did perhaps over-sell the benefits of vitamin C, which he proposed as a cure for cancer and the common cold. Pauling not only used quantum mechanics to understand how atoms in molecules were joined together but also took it upon himself to develop the use of X-ray techniques to understand the structure of the proteins that make up your body. In the process, he was the first to identify the root cause of a genetic disease. He showed that sickle-cell disease occurred because the structure of hemoglobin in people with the disease is slightly different from that of normal hemoglobin. This anomaly was later traced to one difference in the genetic code for hemoglobin in people with sickle-cell disease, which leads to one difference in the amino-acid composition of hemoglobin. This difference produces a hemoglobin molecule that tends to crystallize within blood cells, causing them to adopt a sickle shape, which has many unpleasant consequences, such as an enhanced tendency for stroke as well as priapism—erections that won't go away.

The concept that differences in protein structure, which arise as a result of mutations in your DNA, can cause disease is essential to understanding the importance of a personalized approach to medicine. Protein structure determines ways that you differ from everybody else. If a mutation creeps into your genome that leads to a slightly different structure for a protein, serious genetic diseases can result. For example, individuals who have cystic fibrosis have mutations in their DNA that lead to missing components—and an ineffective structure—in a protein that transports chloride ions across cell membranes. This leads to salty skin, buildup of mucus in the lungs, and other, more serious problems. One in 200 people have genetic mutations that lead to structural defects in proteins that pump ions across the membranes of your heart cells,[3] causing your heart to beat irregularly. Sometimes the first evidence that you have of these mutations is sudden death, so it's important to know if you carry that gene before you die at age nineteen after a particularly intensive session on the basketball court.

X-ray technology also allowed James Watson and Francis Crick (with the considerable assistance of Maurice Wilkins and Rosalind Franklin) to unlock the structure of DNA, revealing the iconic double-helix structure for the first time. This achievement was a culmination of the discoveries of Darwin and the technology made possible by Newton, and it set the path for fifty years of research that would lead to the beginnings of personalized medicine. In research published in 1954, Watson and Crick showed that the structure of DNA led to a logical method by which the sequence of the four "bases" that make up DNA could code for the proteins that do all the work in your body. During a celebration of this discovery at the Eagle Pub in Cambridge, Crick is reported to have exclaimed, "We have discovered the secret of life!" And he was right. To make that relevant to you, however, to unravel the secrets in your genome, methods of determining the sequence of your DNA and proteins it codes for are needed.

Sequencing began with the genius of Fred Sanger, who worked in Cambridge all his professional life, first at the Department of Biochemistry of the University of Cambridge and then the Laboratory of Molecular Biology of the Medical Research Council. It was his genius, as it is with most geniuses, to recognize the obvious. In his case, the obvious was that if proteins do all the work and if the structure of proteins determines how they do that work, it was pretty important to develop ways to discover the sequence of proteins to understand the molecular composition that determines their structure and, therefore, their function. Having solved this problem and won one Nobel Prize, he did the next obvious thing, which was to say that if the sequence of proteins is determined by the sequence of the DNA that codes for the proteins, it was pretty important to sequence DNA too. So he did that as well and won a second Nobel Prize. Thus was born the science of sequencing, which has grown increasingly, unbelievably rapidly over the last twenty years. In 2000, it took ten years and cost $3 billion to complete the first sequencing of a human genome. Now it costs around $1,000 and takes a day or two.[4]

Our ability to measure everything else has grown at equal speed. There are thousands—probably more than 10,000—proteins in your blood. Many of these originate from your brain, your heart, and other organs in your body, and measuring their levels in your blood can potentially diagnose the health of the organ they came from. A technique called mass spectrometry can now be used to rapidly determine the levels of hundreds of different proteins in a drop of blood. The same sequencing techniques used to decode your genome can be applied to characterize the different bacteria in your body by rapidly sequencing the bacterial DNA to determine which bacteria are present. These are the fundamental advances that have given rise to personalized medicine: suddenly we have the ability to measure what you are made of, at the molecular level, for the first time in human history. Contained in all this information are "biomarkers" that are diagnostic for every facet of your being, including what your risks of disease are, what diseases you may actually have, and what diseases you may be trending towards.

Soon, within five years or probably less, all these tests will be available for you as a consumer to buy and use. It is likely that the cost will be less than $100 for each molecular profile, and you will have far more reliable data about yourself than anybody has ever had before. Properly interpreted, this data will provide accurate information about what may be wrong with you and provide strong clues as to how to put it right. Magical thinking will reign no more.

3

THE
MOLECULAR
YOU

AS A RESULT of the efforts of Newton and Maxwell and Darwin and a legion of other scientists and clinicians, we now have the ability to measure a lot about ourselves, not just at the level of organs such as our heart or lungs, not just at the level of the cells that make up the organs and tissues in our bodies, but now at the level of the molecules that make up our cells. These molecules are the most basic determinants of our identities. It is this amazing advance that is fueling the personalized medicine revolution.

Knowledge of yourself at the molecular level is going to have a huge impact on you because you have a fundamental problem. When you were born, you were given a unique body, possibly the most complicated organism on the planet, but you were not given an operator's manual. To use a car as a metaphor, you were not even given very many instruments to monitor how well your body is functioning, and you weren't given any information on the best fuel you should feed your body, whether it should be premium or regular, or whether ethanol can be used as an additive. A number of us seem to run quite well on ethanol, also known as alcohol; but others, not so much. You weren't given any early warning lights to tell you that a life-threatening disease is starting somewhere in your body or that your immune system is going off-kilter, or that some behavior or environmental exposure will lead to arthritis in the future. You have no instrumentation to tell you whether any of those lifestyle changes you make to better your health actually work, and you are usually not quite sure whether the medication you take to fix your aches and pains is doing what it is supposed to do.

In addition to the lack of an operator's manual, you have another, possibly even more basic, problem. Evolution, which led to the exquisitely designed body you live in, does not care about you. Once you are born, you are on your own. If you have lots of children that survive, your genetic code will survive and prosper, but once you have passed child-bearing age, evolution has no further use for the rest of you at all, and your body gradually breaks down and dies. So not only do you need an operator's manual, but you also need to understand how you were made in the first place in order to combat this inevitable decline.

Molecularly based, personalized medicine will give you a rather intimidating operator's manual. It will contain information you may not want to know but really need to be aware of to maintain your health and avoid illness. When used in combination with our ever-improving ability to engineer biological systems, it will provide knowledge that could lead to an ability to fix yourself—your personal repair manual—by manipulating yourself at the cellular and molecular level. It will be by far the most valuable thing you will ever own.

How will we bring your personal operator's manual into reality? The first step is to make an inventory of the molecules that you are made of. The sum total of all this molecular information can be called the "molecular you." The second step is to store all this molecular information in digital form. The resulting dataset comprises the "digital you." The digital version of you will be an impressive amount of data, but not that much use to you unless you can use it to answer your questions about yourself. So the final step on the way to achieving your personal operator's manual will be to devise computerized methods to query your digital self to get definitive answers to important questions you may have.

What questions will your personal manual be able to answer? As we shall see, when fully operational, it will answer more questions than you might think possible. If you don't feel well, you will be able to ask it what is wrong with you and what the best treatment may be. You will be able to find out what drug will most effectively treat whatever disorder you have, and whether you will experience harmful side effects. You will get answers concerning what diet may be best for you and what foods you should avoid. You will be able to find out whether the medicine you're taking or the lifestyle change you've made is effective. It will tell you of your risks of diseases, and you'll get early warnings that a disease is forming in some part of your body well before it becomes life threatening.

The initial versions of your digital self will contain four categories of molecular information, and you can expect more categories to be added over time. First will be your genome: the molecular information that will be measured and stored will be the sequence of your genome, which contains the blueprint of your physical being. Your genome can be taken from almost any cell in your body, as they all contain the same sequence of DNA. Second will be your proteome. Initial measures of your proteome will likely involve determining the levels of 100 or more proteins in your blood, which should be sufficient to get an immediate snapshot of your health. Third will be your metabolome; measurement of 100 or more metabolites in your blood will yield clues as to how your body is dealing with your diet and can also diagnose disease. Finally, we will have to get a measure of your microbiome, or the bacteria and other micro-organisms that live in and on your body. Here, the detection of a few hundred bacteria in your feces will provide vital diagnostic and therapeutic information, particularly for the origin and treatment of immune disorders.

To understand the type of information the digital version of you will provide, and the insight it will give into how to fix whatever is wrong with you, you need to understand a bit about the biology of your body, the processes that go on inside you that make you the fascinating organism that you are. Let's start with your cells—those little bits of you that Leeuwenhoek was the first to observe. You have a lot of cells in your body, approximately 30,000 billion of them, and each of those cells is on average 10 micrometers, or 10 millionths of a meter in diameter. To understand how small a micrometer is, the thickness of the lines forming the letters you're looking at as you read this book is about 100 micrometers. That means ten cells could fit into a line wide enough to be part of a letter big enough for you to read. But the journey towards smallness doesn't end there. Each cell in your body contains a lot of even smaller bits and pieces. Some of these are a thousand times smaller than a cell.

To describe how big these components are, we have to use the nanometer as a measure. There are a thousand nanometers in a micrometer. Luckily, we don't have to go any smaller than that or we'd have to use quantum mechanics to understand ourselves. Each cell contains a nucleus that is approximately 100 nanometers in diameter. And the nucleus contains your genome, your deoxyribonucleic acid, or DNA—the genetic material that codes for the proteins that make the cells that make up your body—wrapped up in twenty-three pairs of bundles called chromosomes. DNA is made of four molecules—guanine (G), cytosine (C), adenine (A), and thymine (T)—known as "bases," which are joined together in long strands. Each of these strands is associated with another "complementary" strand to make up the iconic double-helix structure that Watson and Crick first identified. The complementary strand has a sequence of bases that is complementary to the sequence on the first strand: all the Gs are opposite (paired with) Cs, and all the As are paired with Ts. And vice-versa.

Approximately 99.9 percent of the 3 billion base pairs in your genome are the same as in any other member of the human race. All your differences—the features that make you unique—are encoded by only 0.1 percent of your DNA. But 0.1 percent of your genome corresponds to 3 million base pairs, so there is the potential for a lot of genetic differences. Included in these differences are some sixty brand new mutations— changes in the sequence of bases in your DNA—that have never existed in any person ever before. You really are a mutant. All these genetic differences determine not only differences in eye and hair color between you and anybody else, but also whether you have a higher risk of lung cancer or a lower risk of Alzheimer's disease or a greater chance of a heart attack. The ways that you differ genetically from everybody else also allow the forces of natural selection to work. If you prosper and have lots of children that survive, your genetic code will be conserved and passed down to future generations.

In our exploration of your biology and how molecular-level information such as the sequence of your genome can be incredibly useful, let's start from the beginning, from when your mother and father had (hopefully) a mind-blowing sexual encounter that led to one of your father's sperm cells getting together with one of your mother's eggs to produce a fertilized egg—otherwise known as a totipotent stem cell—from which all the other cells in your body have been made. The sum total of all the DNA in this totipotent stem cell, half of which came from your mother and half from your father, is your genome. The sequence of your genome is fixed: it doesn't change in your lifetime. This DNA supplied all the information needed for the totipotent stem cell to divide time and time again to ultimately form your heart, arms, legs, and every other part of your body. If we could understand all the instructions encoded in your genome, we could predict a lot of things about you: what you would look like at various ages, what reasoning abilities you were going to have—and what diseases you might be susceptible to. Your genome codes for how tall you are, what color eyes you have, how well coordinated you are, the color of your skin—all the physical characteristics you have—whereas your environment has determined what languages you've learned, what religion you might or might not believe in, and which football team is clearly the best in the world as far as you're concerned.

The proteins that your genome codes for enable you to think or move or see or smell. If you had a lethal dose of radiation, which would destroy your DNA, you would not die immediately, but you would be a dead man—or woman—walking. That's because you wouldn't be able to make new proteins to replace old ones as they are degraded; all the proteins in your body are turned over on a regular basis. The sequence of bases in your DNA code for proteins using twenty amino acids that can be put together in any order. It takes a sequence of three bases to code for a particular amino acid, so if a protein is composed of 1,000 amino acids, it requires a gene consisting of a stretch of 3,000 bases of DNA to code for it. In order to make the protein that the gene codes for, the sequence of bases on the gene in the genome is first copied into another stretch of nucleic acids called ribonucleic acid (RNA; which is very similar to DNA) that then contains the code for just this one gene. This "messenger" RNA (mRNA) is then translated into a protein.

The process of forming a protein from a gene is called gene expression. Gene expression and how well the protein produced will work depend on many factors. For instance, gene expression depends on which variant of a gene you've inherited from your parents. These variants can be dominant or recessive, and you need only one copy of a dominant variant—for example, the one that codes for wet earwax—for that trait to be expressed. In contrast, you need two copies of a recessive variant—the one that codes for dry earwax, say, to see that trait expressed.

Lots of things can go wrong with gene expression. If one of the DNA bases in the gene that is expressed is wrong or is omitted, the resulting protein will have a different amino-acid composition and may be defective, leading to genetic diseases such as familial hypercholesterolemia, Huntington's disease, or sickle-cell anemia. The story surrounding the severe form of familial hypercholesterolemia, in which two recessive variants are present, is a great example of how a genetic analysis can lead to basic understanding of a disease and the development of appropriate medicines. Individuals afflicted with severe familial hypercholesterolemia inherit defective genes from both parents that code for a protein called low-density lipoprotein receptor (LDL-R). The cells of these people are unable to accumulate low-density lipoproteins (LDL, commonly referred to as "bad" cholesterol), which transport cholesterol from your liver to peripheral tissues such as muscle and heart. As a result, LDL levels in the blood build to extremely high levels, resulting in cholesterol deposits forming atherosclerotic plaques within the arteries, which then restrict blood flow and cause heart attacks. For people with familial hypercholesterolemia, these heart attacks can occur early in life—during the teenage or young adult years. In families suffering from this condition, there are tales of fathers play-wrestling with their teenage sons, and both father and son dropping dead of heart attacks as a result of the sudden exertion.

In the 1970s, after high cholesterol levels in the blood were identified as the cause of atherosclerosis and high rates of heart attacks, researchers immediately focused on finding ways to inhibit the production of cholesterol in the body to reduce atherosclerosis, which was then the major cause of death in the Western world. This research resulted in the discovery of statins, which interfere with the production of cholesterol in the body. Despite the side effects that statins can have for some people, they have been instrumental in reducing the incidence of heart disease in the Western world to the extent that cancer is now the dominant killer.

Aside from differences in DNA sequence, there are other ways in which protein production can be affected. One common way in which you may differ from the person next to you is in the number of copies of a particular gene you have in your genome. These genetic differences, known as copy number variants (CNVs), can cause changes in the number of proteins made. If you have more copies of a gene that makes proteins that metabolize certain drugs, you will have a different response to those drugs than a "normal" person might. This idiosyncrasy will be revealed when your genome is sequenced. CNVs have also played an important role in evolution. Chimpanzees, for example, make only two copies of a protein known as amylase, which is present in saliva and plays a role in digesting starches, such as those found in potatoes and wheat. Humans, however, can have as many as fifteen copies of amylase—presumably an adaptation that assisted in our transition to a diet that included starchy foods.

A protein that has the wrong amino-acid composition, whether as a result of a faulty gene or errors in either transcription from the genome or translation of the mRNA, probably won't fold into a functional shape. In addition, misfolded proteins are typically not water soluble. An example is the denatured proteins that form the skin on the surface of boiled milk. Misfolded, insoluble proteins in your body can build up as harmful deposits called amyloid plaques and are associated with more than twenty serious human diseases, particularly neurological diseases such as Alzheimer's, Parkinson's, and Huntington's. Amyloid plaques also play a role in prion diseases such as mad cow disease or its inherited human variant, Creutzfeldt-Jakob disease. Once you know which protein is present in the amyloid plaques, you can then design therapies to specifically inhibit production of the protein being deposited, or ways to dissolve the plaque itself.

Only about 2 percent of your genome consists of the 20,000 genes that code for the proteins that make up your body. For a time, it was thought that the "noncoding" regions represented genetic material acquired during human evolution that was no longer needed. Some called these regions "junk DNA."[1] Whoever came up with that phrase should have known better. Evolutionary forces certainly do not favor wasting energy, and it takes a lot of energy to make the enormous amounts of DNA present in the genome in each cell in your body. It turns out that at least some of the noncoding DNA in your genome codes for RNA sequences that do not make proteins but instead regulate gene expression by a process called RNA interference, or RNAi. The RNAi sequences, called microRNA (miRNA) do this by binding to specific mRNA molecules that have a complementary sequence to them. This process causes the mRNA to be degraded and prevents it from making a protein.

MicroRNAs play extensive roles in regulating gene expression in your body, particularly during generation of your organs in embryo, as well as during tissue regeneration and aging. MicroRNAs also play important roles in the growth of cancer cells, and the detection of specific miRNAs in your blood can be diagnostic for the presence of cancer in your body.

All of your cells contain the same genomic DNA, so how do all of the specialized cell types in your body arise? This phenomena is the subject of epigenetics, which concerns how gene expression is regulated so that in specialized cells, only part of the DNA in your genome is translated into proteins. The whole process of differentiation—cells dividing time and time again to form the different organs that you're made of—relies on a highly orchestrated process of genes turning on and off until the subset of proteins that a cell makes are appropriate to its function. For example, muscle cells make lots of long string-like proteins called actin and myosin. Signals transmitted from your brain can cause these proteins to contract, giving rise to muscle movement. In your eyes, large amounts of a protein called rhodopsin are made. Rhodopsin changes its structure when it absorbs light of certain frequencies, and eye cells use this change in structure to transmit a signal to the brain so that you can see. Cell differentiation occurs in a precise fashion. You certainly don't want teeth to form in your muscles or an eyeball to form in your liver.

There are two main ways that a cell can modulate gene expression via epigenetics. There is an on-off switch called methylation, which involves chemically modifying genomic DNA to prevent a gene from being expressed. Alternatively, gene expression can be regulated by controlling how tightly the DNA containing the gene is wound up in the chromosome it is associated with.

Scientists are increasingly able to reverse the differentiation process of a cell to cause it to revert to the stem cells from which the tissue was made.[2] This finding has huge implications for personalized therapeutics and arises from research that has been progressing steadily for more than forty years. In the 1960s, scientists discovered that when the nucleus of a frog skin cell was injected into a frog egg cell whose nucleus had been removed, the recipient egg could produce a normal tadpole. This result means that all the epigenetic controls on the fully differentiated, non-embryonic skin-cell genomic DNA were removed when placed in the environment of the frog egg, indicating that the chemical modifications of the DNA and how tightly it was coiled are reversible. What was also novel and scary was that the new tadpole matured into a new frog that was genetically identical to the frog from which the donor nucleus was derived.[3] This process is called cloning, a graphic example of what was once science fiction coming to life.

Approximately twenty species, ranging from mouse to mule, to horse, to water buffalo, have now been cloned. The first mammal to be cloned was Dolly the sheep.[4] She was cloned in 1996 using cells taken from a donor sheep's udder. As with the frog in the example above, the nucleus was removed from the donor cells and placed in a sheep egg cell from which the nucleus had been removed. The reconstituted egg cell was then placed in the uterus of a host sheep, and Dolly was delivered approximately five months later. She was named Dolly after Dolly Parton because she'd been cloned from udder cells. Who says scientists don't have a sense of humor?

There is little doubt that any human, including you, could be cloned using technology now available. But from a personalized medicine point of view—ethical questions aside—what use would this be to you? It would take years for your clone to be big enough to provide donor organs such as a replacement heart. Apart from the fact that you may not be able to wait that long, by that time your clone may not be too amenable to giving his or her body parts away. It is here that stem cells come to the rescue, at least potentially. You began as a totipotent stem cell that divided to form other cells that, in turn, eventually formed all the other differentiated cells that make up your skin, heart, brain, and so on. All these tissues are renewed regularly: your skin is replaced every two or three weeks, your blood every four months, your skeleton every ten years, and your heart every twenty years. This renewal is orchestrated by "adult" stem cells—that is, cells that are capable of dividing to renew the tissues in which they reside.

So now we have a somewhat less ethically challenged potential solution to renewing failing organs. If you want to renew your heart cells, you need to stimulate, or replace, the adult stem cells that make heart tissue. The same is true for your kidney or any other cells or organs in your body. As a result, stem cells are the subject of intense research, and new findings come daily. Scientists are now working on ways of making stem cells from any tissue by reversing the epigenetic process that leads to the fully differentiated cells, thereby producing "induced pluripotent stem cells (IPSCs)." These IPSCs can then be led back down the differentiation pathway to produce any tissue you may want. For example, skin cells can potentially be reprogrammed to become heart cells. From a personalized medicine standpoint, if, say, you want to see what effect drugs to treat atrial fibrillation will have on your heart as opposed to anyone else's, you should, in the not too distant future, be able to scrape a few cells off the inside of your cheek and get them reprogrammed into cardiac cells that are genetically identical to the ones in your heart. You could then treat them with drugs and drug combinations to determine which ones will work best for you and have the least chance of causing adverse drug reactions.

The future of stem cells as therapeutics is remarkable, given their potential ability to renew any part of your body. One issue is that as you age, the number of adult stem cells in your tissues decreases and their ability to differentiate into functional cells declines. Thus, even though your skin replaces itself every two weeks or so, the new skin produced is not quite as good as the old skin, leading to the thinner, wrinkled skin that older people don't like very much. If we could find a way of stimulating production of adult stem cells in your body, or reprogram them so that they differentiate more accurately, then they could replace your skin with younger skin, your heart with a younger heart, and your bones with younger bones.

While this may seem impossible, do not underestimate the power of the technologies that Newton and Darwin unleashed on the world. Already there are indications that stem cells can be reprogrammed in the tissues where they are found. In an experiment that has connotations of Dracula, researchers at the Harvard Stem Cell Institute connected the circulation of a young mouse to that of an old mouse whose heart was showing signs of hypertrophy, or enlargement, which comes with age and is a precursor to heart failure.[5] Within four weeks of sharing the younger mouse's blood supply, the heart of the older mouse started to become smaller and "younger." A protein, GDF11, which is found in large amounts in young mice but which declines with age, was identified as a possible signal. Sure enough, injection of this protein into older mice produced the same signs of reversed aging in the heart.

So, where are we as we delve down into the molecular you? So far, we have covered how your genome leads to your proteome and the ways that the cell you started from can give rise to all the other cells in your body. But there's a lot more to you than that. There's the old saying "You are what you eat," and in a literal sense, that's true. The proteins, carbohydrates, fats, minerals, and vitamins that you eat all go into making you what you are. A large proportion are either incorporated into proteins in your body or used for energy to power your body. The way that the proteins, carbohydrates, and fats that you eat are used or "metabolized" gives rise to an enormous number of molecules in your body. These molecules are commonly referred to as metabolites.

Consider what happens to proteins, such as those in meat, cheese, or eggs, after you've chewed and swallowed them. They travel to your stomach, where they are bathed in strong acid and are partially decomposed into their constituent amino acids, and then they move into your intestines, where the breakdown is completed. The amino acids that made up the proteins are then transported across the lining of your intestines to enter the bloodstream, where they are taken up by the cells in your body and made into proteins required for cell function. All these amino acids and amino-acid fragments in your blood are metabolites, and the sum total of all the metabolites in your body is your metabolome. If you have defects in your ability to metabolize certain foods, or if you suffer from metabolic diseases such as diabetes, those conditions will be reflected in your metabolome.

You are probably beginning to think, "My God, does this process never end? Do I have to know about every molecule and cell in my body?" Luckily, not really. But if you want to know what data your individualized operator's manual will use to tell you things you really need to know, and also how that information will suggest ways to fix any problems you have, you should stick with the program for just a little longer. There's one more category of things that you're composed of that just has to be included in the molecular description of you: your microbiome—all the bugs that live in and on your body.

Your body is a symbiosis of your human cells with hundreds of trillions of other organisms (microbes) that live inside you and on you. For every one of your cells containing your DNA, you also have ten bacterial cells, and they, along with yeasts, viruses, and parasites, make up your microbiome, which contributes to your state of health in ways we are just beginning to understand. There are more than 10,000 species of bacteria in your body, and these populations differ substantially between individuals. There's a good chance that there are species of bacteria and fungi living inside your ear or in your colon that have not been characterized yet, because many of these organisms have not been grown outside your body. The particular environment in your body that allows them to thrive can be difficult to reproduce.

Bacteria in your microbiome can have a very direct effect on your health. For example, your microbiome possesses most of the gene processing power in your body and can metabolize certain prescription drugs. Thus the makeup of your microbiome can influence the effect drugs have on you. Your microbiome can affect your health in other interesting ways: for example, a *New Yorker* article in 2012 described a man in Pittsburgh who had been suffering for years from a chronic infection in his left ear.[6] His doctors had tried everything, including several types of antibiotics, as well as antifungal drops. Then one day he turned up in the clinic with his ear completely cured of any infection. It turned out that he had taken some of the wax out of his good ear and put it into his bad ear. A few days later, he was fine. Presumably, the bacteria in his good ear had replaced the bacteria that were causing the chronic infection in his bad ear.

A recent review in *Nature* has pointed out the importance of mammals passing through their mother's vagina, which is colonized by an enormous number of types of bacteria.[7] Babies born by Cesarean section do not necessarily pick up these bacteria and may have an incomplete microbiome, which in turn can influence how the baby's immune system develops. In 2012, approximately 30 percent of all children born in North America were born by C-section, and the incidence of allergies and asthma is far higher among those children than it is for vaginal-birth babies.

And it doesn't stop there. It has been some time since it was discovered that the bacterium called *Helicobacter pylori* plays a causative role in the formation of stomach ulcers, leading to the treatment of stomach ulcers by using antibiotics. But why is *H. pylori* there in the first place, and does it play any positive role? The answer would appear to be yes: there is strong evidence that destroying *H. pylori* can alter metabolism in ways that increase the risk of obesity. In people whose stomachs are infected with *H. pylori*, appetite-stimulating hormones are much less detectable after a meal. But in people whose stomachs are not infected, the levels of the hormone remain high, so the message to stop eating doesn't make it to the brain.[8] Research has shown that mice fed antibiotics at dosages similar to those used to treat children with ear infections gained considerable weight compared to mice that did not receive the antibiotic.[9] This, perhaps, is not surprising: most antibiotics consumed in North America are used as dietary supplements to promote faster growth in poultry, cows, and pigs.

We have had a preoccupation with killing bugs since Louis Pasteur showed that infections and illnesses could be caused by microscopic germs entering the body and since Alexander Fleming developed the wonder drug penicillin, which revolutionized our treatment of infectious disease by killing infectious bacteria. However, we may be overdoing it. Perturbing your microbiome by taking antibiotics is not without its dangers. As many as 40 percent of children treated with a broad-spectrum antibiotic will develop a condition called pediatric antibiotic-associated diarrhea due to the havoc that these drugs cause in the bacteria colonizing the intestines.[10] About 10 percent of people carry a dangerous bacterium called *Clostridium difficile*. The bacterium is normally held in check by other residents of the gut. But when those companion bacteria are destroyed by antibiotics, *C. difficile* can erupt, causing severe diarrhea and deadly inflammation in the colon. The infection causes hundreds of thousands of illnesses and 14,000 deaths in America each year. Nearly every *C. difficile* infection occurs as a result of antibiotic treatment.[11]

Conversely, restoring your microbiome to a healthy state by using some rather unusual approaches can dramatically improve your health. For example, fecal transplants replace "bad" bacteria in the gut—those that are associated with diseases such as inflammatory bowel disease—with "good" bacteria taken from healthy donors. The donor's fecal material is placed in the patient's intestines, usually during a colonoscopy. Results from initial clinical trials have been remarkable. In one study to treat inflammatory bowel diseases such as Crohn's disease and ulcerative colitis, sixty patients who were treated using a fecal transplant achieved a 95 percent cure rate. Other trials have reported success rates of more than 80 percent.[12] This is important: nearly a million Americans suffer from inflammatory bowel disease with major effects on their quality of life. Luckily, it is fairly easy to persuade donors for fecal transplants to provide the necessary material, although the recipients may feel less enthusiastic.

The microbiome in your stomach and intestines break down food that your own proteins can't, and in the process, they create vital molecules such as vitamin B and vitamin K. And healthy microbiota in the gut and on the skin, not to mention in the ears, eyes, and respiratory and reproductive systems, can be allies against infections by harmful bacteria. Striking the right microbial balance is key: for example, the vagina is home to yeasts and bacteria that usually keep each other in check. A subtle change to the vaginal environment can cause one population to flourish over another, resulting in a yeast infection.

So the molecular version of you has to include your personal microbiome. You will have to get over any squeamishness you may have about the bugs that live symbiotically with you; they are a vital part of your being. You are a tightly coordinated system consisting of billions of micromachines and nanomachines, all of which have to run smoothly individually and act together to produce the living, breathing you.

If the thought of fecal transplants and borrowed earwax to rescue your microbiome seems a little weird or possibly abhorrent to you, you're not the only one. It points to a possible problem in Western society: in our quest for cleanliness, we may have gone overboard. Many immunological and autoimmune disorders are much less common in the third world than they are in the Western world. Almost 10 percent of youth in North America suffer from asthma, but in rural Africa it is much less prevalent. This situation may be related to a need to keep your immune system healthy by challenging it appropriately.

Realizing how complicated your immune system is and getting a little dirty may be an important component of your personalized medicine protocol. For example, certain immune cells contain components called toll-like receptors (TLRs) that help to fend off infectious agents. There are more than ten TLRs present in immune cells in the skin and other places susceptible to infection, and TLRs are quite specific with regard to the type of bug that they are programmed to react to and destroy. TLR3, TLR8, and TLR9 recognize RNA from viruses. Most others are specific for proteins found in bacteria. What is clear is that inappropriate activation of these receptors leads to autoimmune problems. Artificial activation of TLR4, for example, which is programmed to respond to certain bacterial infections, gives rise to asthmatic symptoms.

Given the fact that your immune system has evolved to protect you against bacterial and other infections, and that you contain such an enormous population of bacteria and other microbes, it should come as no surprise that your microbiome can have major effects on the function of your immune system. Your microbiome and immune system are clearly barely tolerant of each other, yet they are dependent on each other. Scientists recently demonstrated that the immune systems in genetically identical, same-sex mice responded quite differently to the same stimuli. This effect was eventually traced to different microbiome compositions in the individual mice. So disorders of your immune system, which range from asthma to arthritis, to inflammatory bowel disease, can potentially originate from, or be exacerbated by, an imbalanced microbiome.

The very presence of organisms that the immune system was evolved to fight may be necessary for proper immune function. The lack of stimulation of our immune system in early life and the development of immunological problems later on has led to the "hygiene hypothesis": that clean upbringings, relatively free of parasites and infectious agents, do not lead to development of a healthy immune system and can cause it instead to become hyperactive. A hyperactive immune system is not what you want: it can result in everything from allergies to disorders in which your immune system attacks your own tissues, such as occurs in multiple sclerosis or lupus.

Keeping your immune system occupied in fighting the battles it was designed to fight might just reduce the chances of it becoming oversensitive and starting to reject parts of you. People who are infected with hookworms seem to suffer fewer autoimmune-related diseases, including asthma and hay fever. This observation has led to a fairly radical treatment for auto-immune disorders known as Helminthic therapy. This sounds innocuous enough until you realize that it involves infecting yourself with parasitic worms that your immune system evolved to fight many eons ago. Helminthic therapy has been proposed as a treatment for a variety of autoimmune diseases: inflammatory bowel disease, multiple sclerosis (a nasty autoimmune disease affecting 300,000 North Americans, in which the body attacks the insulation surrounding its own neurons), asthma, dermatitis, and food allergies.[13]

Although maintaining your microbiome in a healthy state and in balance with your immune system appears to be a good idea, there is certainly good reason not to go all the way with getting dirty again. The health gains made by the development and use of antibiotics and vaccines are enormous. However, eating a little dirt, avoiding antibiotics when you can, and getting a few infections, especially when you're young, may not be a bad thing either. While we are still a long way from a detailed understanding of the relationship between your microbiome and your health, the outline is becoming clear. We have evolved an immune system to deal with bugs and parasites of all sorts, resulting in a curious symbiosis and a delicate balance. If your microbiome is perturbed, you will be too.

The catch phrase for an old detective TV series called *Dragnet* was "Just the facts, ma'am, just the facts"; and in this chapter, we have covered a lot of facts regarding the things that make up the molecular you. And your genome, your proteome, your metabolome, and your microbiome are just the start. There are other "omes" that have not been mentioned and more yet to be discovered. Hidden in this treasure trove of molecular information are facts that provide the clues vital to the detective work of finding out what is right or wrong with you; whether you are in the early stages of disease and whether the therapy you are undergoing is working. So now we have to find ways of measuring all these molecules to get a description of you at a molecular level, put it into digital form, and then figure out what it means. That's the topic of the next chapter.

4

THE
DIGITAL
YOU

BY NOW, YOU might be asking, "If personalized medicine is so important, where is it? My doctor has never mentioned it. I read this abstract stuff in the paper or in magazines saying new genetic tests will bring us to a cure for cancer in five years or whatever, but people have been saying stuff like that for twenty years. As far as I can see, medicine hasn't really changed that much in my lifetime. It still seems pretty hit or miss." The unfortunate thing is, you're absolutely right.

But this time it's different.

What makes personalized medicine possible now is described by that overused term convergence. A multitude of technologies have now begun to converge to make personalized medicine possible. The technologies that originated with Newton and Darwin now provide us with the ability to sequence your genome from, say, one of your skin cells in a couple of hours, measure a few hundred proteins or metabolites from a drop of your blood to characterize your proteome and metabolome, or describe the microbiome you never wanted to know you had by analyzing fecal matter taken from toilet paper you have just used. There's the computer technology originated by Babbage and Turing and enabled by the nanotechnology envisioned by Feynman, all of which gives us the enormous data storage and processing power that we need to deal with the massive data cloud consisting of your genome, your proteome, your metabolome, and your microbiome; the sum total of which describes you more completely than anything ever has before. Then there's the technology originated by Maxwell that led to the electronic age, the Internet, social media, and all the remote-sensing devices that are now available. All of these technologies are converging to measure you at the molecular level, store these data digitally, analyze this "digital you" to determine your state of health and disease and then suggest the best way to keep you in a healthy state or treat any illness diagnosed.

The concept of the digital you is very important, though you may find it unsettling that such detailed information about you should be rendered in such an accessible form. But that ability is just another expression of the digital revolution, otherwise known as the information age, which in two short generations has transformed almost everything in our civilization. Except medicine. We used to have typewriters; now we have computers. We used to write letters; now we email. We used to go to the library if we wanted to find something out; now we use Google. We used to have travel agents; now we have Expedia. We used to have phones that weren't all that smart and that stayed in one place; now we have portable phones that can do more than we can comprehend. We used to have records and record players and more recently compact discs, and they too are going the way of the dodo as smartphones and cloud services become music central. There are many other industries in transition. We still have books that are made of paper, but Amazon and Kindle have other intentions. We still have cars that you actually have to drive, but Google will change that soon. The list is endless, but the technology is the same. Everything is being reduced to digital form so that it can be readily stored, transmitted, analyzed, and utilized.

Consider a song. One hundred years ago, if you wanted to hear someone sing a song, you had to take out the horse and buggy or fire up the Model T and go to the theater to hear it. Or you could have bought some rather scratchy recordings that sounded vaguely like the original artist when played on a phonograph, but the effect certainly was not the same. Things improved as vinyl records became available after the Second World War but then changed completely in the 1980s, when compact discs replaced them. So what happened? We moved from analogue to digital. Records and their precursors relied on picking up the sound vibrations from the air and imprinting those vibrations as little ridges in grooves on the wax or plastic surface of a record. If the record was then spun at the right speed, and a needle was placed in the grooves of the record to rub over the ridges, it would vibrate, and you heard the song. That was analogue recording. Digital recording onto a compact disc is completely different. Here, the sound vibrations are converted into a stream of numbers representing the frequency and intensity of sound over time. When placed in a CD player, these numbers are converted back into sounds by reversing the recording process. Now, of course, we are forgetting about the CD and streaming the numbers from the Internet directly to your computer or iPhone to reconstruct the song. Similarly, when we are creating the digital you, we convert your molecular information into numbers that can be used to recreate you—or at least a pretty good imitation of you. It won't quite be you, but it will hum a few bars.

What bars will it hum? Well, initially, it too will be a little scratchy, but the main thing is that you will be able to start asking your digital self some important questions. Your person-alized operator's manual will start to come to life. For example, once you have your genome in a digitized format, you'll be able to ask it whether you will have a bad reaction to a drug that your doctor prescribes, whether that drug will make you cough, or whether it will work on you at all. You'll be able to ask it about your risk of inherited diseases. You may soon be able to ask it whether you have any chance of being that elite athlete you always wanted to be or whether a career as a rocket scien-tist is in the cards. More seriously, if you get cancer, you will be able to have your cancer-cell genome sequenced and ask which mutated genes are present and which drugs may best be used to treat them. The convergence of social media and patient-to-patient organizations could well lead you to post your cancer genome on the Internet so that you can find out what other people with similar cancer genetic profiles have done and how well their therapies have worked for them. This represents a rather interesting transition of power, one in which patients, as opposed to doctors or scientists, get to decide on what informa-tion gets shared with whom.

So far, so good. What else will the digital you enable you to do? A lot more. As you start to monitor your proteome, say, in the form of the proteins in a particular bodily fluid such as your blood, you'll get a lot more data that you can add to your digital self. You'll have to do this regularly, maybe every two or three months, in order to get data showing that you're trend-ing in one direction or another, as your proteome can change substantially depending on your health. If you are trending towards other diseases such as arthritis or diabetes, you will see increases in inflammatory proteins or retinol-binding pro-tein respectively. Seeing these "biomarker" proteins move in the wrong direction may be enough to get you off the couch occasionally. Eventually your proteome will provide early warning of everything from heart failure to kidney failure, to viral infections, lung disease, stroke, heart attacks, cancer— you name it. And when stored in your digital self and looked at over time, you'll be able to see whether you're moving in the right or the wrong direction, and whether the efforts you're making to avoid full-blown disease are working or not. You will be able to experiment with your digital self to see whether your diet, lifestyle change, or exercise program is doing what you want it to.

Your metabolome and your microbiome will also be part of the digital you. Your microbiome may be off-kilter because you have overused antibiotics, your diet is wrong for you, or you inherited an unhealthy variety of bacteria from your mother. You may well want to complement all this information with other data, such as your blood pressure, electrocardiogram, heart rate, and sleeping patterns, as gathered by the recording devices that you wear. Eventually, when we can find ways of measuring it, you will want to store your brain connectome (the connections between neurons in your brain) to get a handle on your mental health and why you feel so irrationally happy, even though your digital you says you shouldn't. Or vice-versa. So the questions now become how do we gather the data we want, how do we store it, and how do we analyze it so that you can get answers to your questions about that most important person: you.

Let's start by sequencing your genome. The DNA-sequencing methods developed by Sanger have now been supplanted by much faster, next-generation sequencing techniques in which the genomic DNA is first broken down into thousands of short fragments. The sequence of each of these fragments is then determined simultaneously using millions of reactions all going on at the same time. The sequences of the DNA fragments are then fed into a database and analyzed by genome-assembly software that relies on finding fragments that contain regions with the same DNA sequence, to reconstruct the sequence of the entire genome. But technology isn't stopping there: new approaches are on the horizon that can sequence DNA through electronic techniques rather than the chemical techniques originated by Sanger. These methods could decrease the time it takes to sequence human genomes to a couple of hours, using a device only slightly bigger than a USB memory stick. In this device, the DNA to be sequenced is fed as long strands through a nanopore—a hole with a diameter of a few nanometers—and the electrical resistance as the bases pass through the hole is measured. Each base has a slightly different size or charge, giving a distinct resistance signature for each base and thus allowing the sequence to be determined.[1]

All this sequencing stuff may sound like science fiction, but think of this: when you were an embryo in your mother's womb, the process of sequencing your genomic DNA and making a new copy in a dividing cell took about five hours. Three billion base pairs were read during that time, and three billion new base pairs made, corresponding to a rate of 160,000 bases per second, all with an error rate of less than one in every 10 million bases that were made.[2] Talk about nanotechnology in action! We don't have to invent any of this, just reverse engineer it. So genome sequencing is certainly going to get even faster, and cheaper, than it is today.

How about proteomics? How are we measuring different proteins, what tissues are we taking the proteins from, and how are the data related to health and disease? Most effort is going into using the blood as a window into what is happening inside us. Your blood bathes every organ in your body, and proteins specific to each of your organs leach out into the blood as it passes through. It has been estimated that we could measure the health of a particular organ by measuring a subset of only twenty or so proteins in the blood that originate from that organ. The problem is that there are many thousands of proteins in the blood and they differ in concentrations by more than nine orders of magnitude.[3] In other words, some proteins are present at concentrations that are more than a billion times higher than other proteins, and this makes the less-prevalent proteins difficult to detect and quantify.

One technique used to measure your proteome is mass spectrometry. Each protein in your blood has a unique molecular weight, and mass spectrometers are very good at detecting the molecular weights of molecules in a sample, from which the identity of the protein the sample contains can be determined. Other techniques use very specific tags such as antibodies or smaller molecules that bind to particular blood proteins very tightly but don't bind to any others. By measuring the amounts of a given molecular tag that is associated with a blood sample, for example, the species and amounts of a given protein in your blood can be determined. Although it is difficult to predict which technique will be the winner, it's clear that we now have the ability to measure many hundreds, if not a thousand, proteins in a blood sample within a few hours and at costs of less than $1,000. Like genomic analyses, proteomic analyses of your blood are going to get faster and cheaper and, in the near future, will no doubt cost less than $100 for measurement of a hundred or more proteins.

At present, blood proteins are analyzed one by one in specialized laboratories, and the results reported to your doctor a week or so later. But the day is fast approaching when a much more complete version of your proteomic profile will be available to you directly for uploading into your digital self. There are a number of ways this could be done. Christoph Borchers of the University of Victoria, for example, has developed mass spectrometry techniques that allow dried blood proteins to be reliably analyzed.[4] To obtain your blood protein profile by this approach, you would simply smear a pinprick of blood on a piece of blotting paper and FedEx it to the laboratory, getting the results back by email to be downloaded into your digital self a couple of days later. Eventually, it is possible that a small, disposable chip will be developed to perform similar functions in real time. Analysis of the proteomic data will reveal immediately useful information, ranging from levels of bad or good cholesterol (no more cheesecake!) to whether the chemotherapy you are taking to treat your cancer is working, whether your cancer has returned, whether you are trending towards a heart attack, whether that hit on the head caused a concussion—in short, a complete snapshot of your health and disease status.

The technique used to measure your microbiome could be the same genome-sequencing technology used to decipher your genomic DNA, but this time samples from your ear, nose, or feces, which contain high levels of bacteria and other microbes, will be analyzed. Rapid genome sequencing of the microbes will detect the presence of particular strains of bacteria and other microbes that coexist with you by detecting their characteristic genetic signatures. The populations detected will depend on where the sample is taken from, as bacterial populations vary substantially based on whether they are taken from your mouth, ear, skin, or stool. Similarly, measurement of your metabolome will depend on whether samples are taken from your urine, blood, saliva, or fecal matter. Here again, the technique will probably be mass spectrometry. Investment in companies that make mass spectrometers would seem to be a good bet as the practice of personalized medicine becomes more prevalent: mass spectrometry has become the go-to technique for the rapid detection of hundreds of different molecules present in biological samples. You are likely already familiar with mass spectrometers: simple versions are used at airports to detect chemicals that indicate the presence of explosives.

Once all this information has been collected, it needs to be stored and analyzed. The problem of storage will probably be easily solved, although some people may tell you otherwise. There will be a lot of data. But all we have to do is wait for a little while, and technology will deal with it—at least, that's the lesson of recent history. The cost of data storage used to be astronomical. In 1956, you would have had to pay $10 million for one gigabyte (a billion bytes) of storage. In 1981, the cost of a gigabyte was $300,000. By the year 2000, it had dropped to $10. In 2010, the price of storing a gigabyte of data dropped to just 10¢.[5] Prices have dropped because technology improved and storage devices can be created at much lower costs. The sizes of the devices that can store the data are also much smaller.

Even so, some people will point out that we're talking about a lot—and here we mean a *lot*—of data. Storing your genome of roughly 3 billion base pairs requires about 800 megabytes of storage. Genes are often sequenced many times to ensure accuracy, so it's common to save approximately 100 gigabytes, or 100,000 megabytes, of information for a single human genome.[6] That amount of data can definitely be costly to store, but there are always ways around problems. For starters, you could store just the differences between your genome and a common reference genome. This tactic reduces things by 99.9 percent. Or you could store a few cells in the refrigerator and re-sequence the genome as needed. At a sequencing cost of $100 or less, this method may well be cheaper than storing the data electronically.

So, you say, "That's good so far, very impressive. I can see how we'll generate all this information and store it, but you still haven't told me how I'm going to use this damn data to prevent or cure my disease or make myself feel better." Ah, yes—slight problem there. That's where the bottleneck is, and any readers who want a well-paid, highly secure occupation for the next twenty years should become experts in bioinformatics, particularly as it pertains to interpreting the large datasets surrounding genomic, proteomic, and other "omic" information. To illustrate some of the difficulties, let's look at cancer treatment. Each cancer cell usually has between twenty and eighty mutations that distinguish it from a normal cell. The question then becomes, which mutated genes are the driver mutations—the mutations that cause the cancer to grow? The cancer bioinformatics community is now tackling problems like this one with some success. However, the fact that a person's cancer may have different mutations depending on which tumor in their body is tested or from where in any given tumor the sample is taken indicates the scale of the problem. Before appropriate therapy can be designed for a particular cancer patient, multiple sequencing of different cancer cells taken from different biopsies from that patient would need to be done.

Nonetheless, you can start to see why personalized medicine is increasingly possible. You can now get some pretty detailed molecular-level information about yourself. And you can store it digitally, either in the cloud or on your own hard drive if you don't like sharing your personal bytes. You can also see how the data you collect about yourself may be useful for detecting genetic diseases and finding new treatments for diseases such as cancer: if we can determine causative genes, we can then try to inhibit them. But personalized medicine is much more useful than that—a fact that will become clear as the digital you is compared with the digital versions of thousands of other people. You're probably familiar with the concept of big data in various contexts, such as the collection of closed-circuit camera surveillance data in a major city. We are getting increasingly adept at mining big data for the information we want. Within days of the London bombings in 2005, facial-recognition software had, from the tapes of hundreds of closed-circuit TVs, identified the bombers. One can only imagine how fast that could be done today. Similar analyses of the big data that will soon be surrounding you, with similar data clouds derived from other people, will reveal enormously interesting information.

So how does comparison of your data with data from other individuals help identify the causes of your disorders and result in a therapy meant just for you? One example concerns the relation between genotype (your genome) and phenotype (your personal traits). Comparison of genotype with phenotype over thousands or millions of individuals will reveal in exquisite detail how various genes contribute to every aspect of you, from the color of your hair to a tendency to lisp to athletic potential. If we analyze a subset of people taking a particular drug, we can start to correlate who'll have symptoms such as dizziness, nausea, fatigue, or other nasty side effects according to their genetic makeup. The correlation between the genotype of people with a particular disease and their environment will start to bring to light the subtle relationship between environment and individual susceptibility to disease.

For people with a particular disease, using social media to compare their digital self with that of many others suffering from the same disorder will have major impact. By correlating the severity of disease and the effectiveness of various therapies with genomic and other "omic" data, we can expect the development of improved, individualized treatments. The impact of social media and the Internet on health is already profound: more than 80 percent of Internet users now use "Dr. Google" to research health-related issues. Virtual communities focused on health and disease are thriving. One such community, PatientsLikeMe, was originally founded to connect people suffering from amyotrophic lateral sclerosis (ALS) with each other but now includes people with hundreds of other conditions, including multiple sclerosis, HIV, and fibromyalgia, and as of early 2014, has more than 220,000 members,[7] providing a forum for patients to share their stories and report on how well the treatments they undergo work for them. The effectiveness of these sites for determining the best therapies will be dramatically amplified when patients start sharing their digital selves with each other.

Even without sharing personal digital data, some of these patient networks already drive new ways to treat disease. The CureTogether network[8] was founded to help people with chronic pain and allows its members to anonymously rate the various treatments they've tried, resulting in what can be characterized as a virtual clinical trial. For instance, members with vestibulodynia, a chronic-pain condition affecting the vulva, were invited to self-report the effectiveness of various treatments over a three-year period. When the pooled data were analyzed, it was found that conventional treatments actually made the condition worse, whereas other therapies were surprisingly helpful. CureTogether now has patient-reported reviews of treatments for arthritis, Crohn's disease, and bipolar disorder, among other conditions. CureTogether was recently acquired by 23andMe, a direct-to-consumer genomic sequencing and analysis company, which will gather genetic information on patients to see how this data relates to effectiveness of treatment and the toxicities associated with various drug therapies.

Patient networks can also enable research efforts to develop new drugs to treat diseases that have no cure. Again, these efforts will gain considerable focus and momentum when patients begin sharing their genomic, proteomic, and other personal data with each other. These networks already have some notable successes; for example, PXE International was founded by Patrick and Sharon Terry in 1995 after their two children were diagnosed with pseudoxanthoma elasticum (PXE), a rare genetic disorder that can cause blindness. PXE International founded a tissue bank to collect samples from PXE patients for genetic analysis to try to find the gene causing PXE.[9] In 1999, using this tissue bank, researchers determined the gene responsible, and a diagnostic test for PXE was developed in 2007. If you know the causative gene for a condition, the search for a treatment is much more straightforward. Many researchers are now engaged in finding a treatment for PXE.

Patient groups and social media also allow other virtual clinical trials to be performed. Knowing that patients suffering from a side effect will try to find information about it online, Russ Altman and colleagues at Stanford University found that patients on the antidepressant Paxil who were also taking the cholesterol-lowering Pravachol (pravastatin) were more likely to search for symptoms of hyperglycemia, or high blood-sugar levels, which include dehydration, blurry vision, or frequent urination. "Historically, it's been really hard to detect synergistic effects of drug combinations that aren't necessarily side effects of any of the drugs alone,"[10] Russ Altman commented. "I believe patients are telling us lots of things about drugs, and we need to figure out ways to listen." This information regarding the interaction of Paxil and Pravachol is important, particularly for people who are already diabetic, as it turned out that their blood-sugar levels were raised substantially if they were taking both of these drugs. Such interactions could potentially be discovered very directly by mining shared digital databanks of patient groups concerned with depression or high blood-cholesterol levels.

So there will be techniques to measure a lot of things about you to construct a digital version of yourself, methods for analyzing that data to relate it to your health, and ways of sharing that data with others to arrive at improved diagnoses and treatments. But it doesn't stop there. All this information is going to be combined with data obtained by technology allowing remote sensing of your physical status. These analyses will provide information about vital signs such as heart rate, respiration, blood pressure, and temperature, in addition to more specialized data. Monitors for blood-glucose levels in diabetics are a particular priority: nearly 10 percent of the population of the United States has diabetes, costing the health-care system an estimated $245 billion every year.[11] Diabetes contributes to the deaths of more than 200,000 people a year and can reduce life span by up to ten years. Much of the damage due to diabetes could be prevented by keeping blood-glucose levels within a narrow range, and many companies are developing sensors to measure glucose levels that report back to an insulin pump, which will administer precisely the right amount of insulin. This process has to be fail-safe, however, as too much insulin can lower blood sugar to levels that result in coma and death, which is the terror of parents of infants with type 1 diabetes.

Many other mobile health devices are in the planning or testing stages. There are already apps for your phone that allow you to perform an electrocardiogram to ascertain the health of your heart. If you're concerned about an irregular rhythm, the graph can be emailed to your doctor. Implantable cardioverter defibrillators, which give the heart a shock when they detect an arrhythmia, are in testing phases. Cardiac bandages to monitor heart function twenty-four hours a day, seven days a week, are now available that transmit directly to your computer. Sensors are under development that can be embedded in a small vein to detect circulating cells that have been sloughed off from weakened blood-vessel walls as much as a week before a heart attack. This research is really important, since approximately half of all heart attacks are fatal, causing nearly 600,000 deaths per year in the U.S. alone.[12] It would be good to have early warning of these events well before you drop dead. Similar embedded devices are in the works that will aid in cancer detection (by detecting cancer cells derived from a primary tumor) or in detection of everything from lupus to celiac disease.

So if you think that you already have enough apps for your smartphone, you are sadly mistaken. The number of apps that will be available to monitor your health will soon constitute a dominant proportion of the market. Aside from receiving messages from sensors on and in your body that will allow you to monitor your health minute by minute (it is hard to imagine the joy this will give a serious hypochondriac or the agony it will cause their doctors), your smartphone will be able to access your digital you to upload new data and to download other data to analyze as needed. You'll certainly be able to access your genomic data at the doctor's office to help him or her decide which drug would be best for you and which you should avoid.

So the digital version of you—which is the sum of your genomic, proteomic, metabolomic, microbiomic, and potentially other omic data, combined with a digital record of your vital signs over time as detected by remote sensing—is on the way. This data will be informative, to say the least—particularly when you compare your digital self with the digital versions of others in your situation. The biggest single gap that remains is interpretation of this data. But as you can see from the progress being made with big data, it will become very precise, very soon.

So, you ask, when can I give this digital version of me a test run? When can I get my hands on my very own operator's manual? The next chapter will show that in many ways, your digital self and operator instructions to get diagnoses based on molecular-level information can be a reality right now. All those questions you're scared to know the answers to will soon be answered. If you want them to be.

5

SIGNS
OF THE
REVOLUTION

THE TIPPING POINT, where medical practice will suddenly adopt the principles of personalized medicine, will be reached within the next five years. You will experience a memorable personal tipping point when you first get your genome sequenced, your microbiome analyzed, your metabolome assayed, and your proteome measured and then sit down with your doctor or wellness coach to discuss the implications of this very definitive data that is all about you. The data will be so precise and all-encompassing that it will show not only what may be wrong with you but also what you ate for breakfast yesterday and what type of dog you own. The impact of this information on you and the way you live your life will be greater than any other technological advance you have ever experienced. Remember when you started using Google and suddenly had access to all the information in the world and couldn't imagine how you operated before? Or, for those who are old enough, remember the feeling you had when you started using email and suddenly had immediate communication with all parts of the world, for free? Or, for those of you who are really old, the first time you realized that having your own computer could actually be useful? Or, for those of you who, like the author, are positively ancient, the time you picked up your first hand-held calculator that could multiply and divide and take square roots? Well the personalized medicine revolution will trump them all.

The harbingers of the revolution are all around us.

Early versions of the digital version of you are starting to appear, although progress has been slow because of the enormous institutional, technical, and societal issues involved. The deeply conservative instincts of the medical profession have not helped either. The first manifestation of the digital you is (or will be) your electronic medical record (EMR) sometimes known as your electronic health record (EHR). The first attempts to introduce EMRs date back to the late 1960s; in the 1970s, the Department of Veterans Affairs had a working Computerized Patient Record System that established the ability of EMRs to reduce medical errors. Problems ranging from lack of standards, security concerns, and aversion to change prevented general adoption of EMRs until, with some frustration, President Obama pushed the Health Information Technology for Economic and Clinical Health Act into law in 2009. The legislation mandated a transition to EMRs for physicians and hospitals that treat patients covered by government insurance.

Still, it is surprising that in the U.S. in 2012 (the latest year for which records are available), only 72 percent of physicians used any form of electronic health record, ranging from just 54 percent in New Jersey to 89 percent in Massachusetts. In 2009, only 48 percent of physicians used EMRs. And right now, EMRs are not all that complicated. They consist of a digital store of your complete medical history, including medications and allergies, immunization status, laboratory test results, radiology images, vital signs, and personal statistics like age and weight. The lack of EMRs has meant untold duplication, errors due to incomprehensible handwriting, lack of knowledge about pre-existing conditions, and ongoing patient frustration with doctors who refuse to enter the digital age that the rest of us embraced twenty years ago. How many times have you been referred to a doctor, only to be asked the same questions all over again or be required to do a test that you've already done, simply because the doctor has no access to an electronic version of your medical history?

Some of the reasons for delay, it has to be admitted, are not the fault of the medical profession. Privacy is an enormous concern. Your EMR, because it is in electronic form, is susceptible to the same sort of hacking as any other personal data stored on your computer or by your credit card company or by your bank. Clearly you don't want an insurer or employer to get hold of your medical record without your authorization. But if your bank can achieve a secure online system for you to conduct your financial transactions, why can't one be created for your medical information? Regardless, the digitization dam that's been holding back universal EMRs has clearly burst, and we are finally entering the digital age of medicine.

Assuming you have one, can you get hold of your own electronic medical record? You should be able to—after all, it's all about you. But ownership can be complicated, and doctors who have purchased an EMR system may feel that information in it about you belongs to them. Often, a strange distinction exists: the doctor or hospital owns your medical record, but you own the data in your medical record. In any event, if your medical record is digitized, you should be able to get hold of a digital copy.

The next step will be to add your genomic, proteomic, microbiomic, and all the other data to your EMR to achieve a more complete digital version of yourself. Early signs of development of such personalized data clouds and their utility are being seen for a small number of individuals who have access to the sophisticated resources currently required in order to study themselves in detail at the molecular level. One example is Michael Snyder, a geneticist at Stanford University. He learned that he was at high risk for developing type 2 diabetes as a result of a genetic analysis.[1] "I was not aware of any type-2 diabetes in my family and had no significant risk factors," Snyder said, "but I learned through genomic sequencing that I have a genetic predisposition to the condition." He decided to study his molecular self using the resources of his laboratory to gather and interpret the data. Over a fourteen-month period, Snyder had his blood drawn twenty times for a proteomic and metabolomic analysis to construct what his research team called his "integrative personal omics profile," or iPOP. During those fourteen months, Snyder contracted two viral infections, and during the second infection, his glucose levels spiked. Snyder was subsequently diagnosed with type 2 diabetes, and in response, he altered his diet and ramped up his exercise routine. After six months, his glucose levels returned to normal without any drug treatment. Knowing that he was predisposed to diabetes allowed him to take immediate action when he saw changes in his blood-glucose levels, bringing the disease to a halt. "This is the first time that anyone has used such detailed information to proactively manage their own health," said Snyder. He added, "Right now, this type of analysis is very expensive. But we have to expect that, like whole-genome sequencing, it will get much cheaper. And we also have to consider the savings to society from preventing disease."

Individuals like Michael Snyder are pointing the way to how medicine of the future will be practiced. It will be much more proactive than reactive; detecting disease at the earliest stages before it becomes too late. It is obvious that not many of us will have access to the resources that Snyder has to either gather the molecular-level data required or to interpret it. However, there are many companies springing up to perform the genomic, protcomic, metabolomic, and microbiomic analyses required. There are now more than twenty companies and institutes worldwide that will sequence your genome for you, including companies such as Illumina in the U.S. and institutes such as the Beijing Genomics Institute (BGI) in China. BGI, which had more than 4,000 employees in 2011 and is presumably considerably larger now, was a key player in the 1,000 genomes project to sequence 1,000 people from a variety of ethnic origins to gain insight into human genetic variation. This data was published in the journal *Nature* in 2012. Companies are being formed on an almost daily basis to conduct proteomic, metabolomic, and microbiomic characterizations as the technology required for high-throughput analyses comes on line.

Interpretation of the resulting datasets will probably be the rate-limiting factor in extending the benefits of these molecular-level examinations to the general population. Much of this interpretation will first be performed by panels of experts in particular diseases, who will analyze the digital records of hundreds or thousands of patients to discover what combination of omic data provides the most accurate diagnostics or suggests the most appropriate therapies for individual patients. It is possible that machine-learning techniques, such as those used by Amazon to suggest books for you based on your purchasing history, will also be employed to detect patterns in the data. Computer algorithms will then be written that will allow these findings to be applied to everybody else.

You or your doctor will use these "expert system" algorithms to analyze your own particular digital data cloud to diagnose disease and to decide on therapy. This new process has major implications. Expert diagnostic and prognostic systems will be continually refined as data from people around the world with similar omic profiles and diseases are analyzed, and such systems will certainly be able to prescribe more reliable, personalized medical advice than your doctor can currently provide. You will still be better off if you have a doctor, but he or she will be of a different sort than the one you have now.

Doctors of the future not only will sit down with you and examine the physical you, but will also have to analyze your digital self with you, bringing to your attention not only the signals of health and disease, but also the latest methods of interpretation, pointing out trends in your biological data that are moving in the wrong direction and helping you find ways to reverse them. Your doctor will have to change from being your disease manager to being your health coach, working with you as part of a team to keep you in an optimal state of health. This kind of relationship is different from the one most of us have with our doctors at the moment.

The first signs of this changing relationship are evident, and not all physicians are happy about it. Many of us are becoming our own doctors: armed with information gleaned from the Internet, we march into the doctor's office with diagnoses of our own conditions. Eighty percent of us use the Internet the instant we feel something is wrong. This phenomenon is leading to terms such as cyberchondria: sufferers obsessively search the 'net for any symptom they may have, invariably finding that they are suffering from a particularly aggressive form of an incurable disease. But Internet research does serve a useful and—for many—essential purpose.

Many of us do not have doctors we can call on, and Dr. Google is our only recourse. For people who do, does anybody have a doctor who has truly joined the digital age? One you can send emails to and set up appointments with electronically? Does anybody have a doctor who has instant access in his or her office to the latest X-ray scans done when you visited the emergency room at a local hospital because of an intestinal complaint? Does anyone have a doctor who scans the latest scientific literature and calls you up when some recent finding may be important for you to know? Not very many of us can answer yes to even the first two questions, which makes doctor's visits sometimes frustrating and Dr. Google very inviting; and nobody has a doctor who is up to date with the scientific literature and who can analyze your digital data to determine what is relevant to you. So right now, if you want to take advantage of the benefits of personalized medicine, you are going to have to start to assemble your digital self yourself as best you can and use your doctor as a sounding board to help interpret what you find. Some people may complain about having to do this, but it is really very empowering. Acquiring your own digital data and using it to answer questions you have about yourself is the first step in demystifying your body in health and disease and constitutes the initial stages of the personalized medicine revolution: you are finally getting the information you need for your very own operator's manual and using it to take care of your own health.

The forces driving this transition are profound. Physicians will say you should always see a doctor before self-medicating, and so you should. It has been estimated that a simple Dr. Google search to correlate your symptoms with a disease results in a correct self-diagnosis 60 percent of the time.[2] Using this information to determine which drug you should take is therefore not a good idea, as 40 percent of the time you'd be wrong. But doctors are often wrong too. It has been estimated that in the U.S., up to 15 percent of doctors' diagnoses of diseases leading to death were proven wrong on autopsy.[3] Diagnosis of your disorder is absolutely key to successful treatment. It is unlikely that you will be cured of pneumonia when the problem is lung cancer.

And here's where the digital you that includes genomic, proteomic, and other molecular data is going to have enormous impact, because when you ask your molecular self what the problem is, your chance of getting the correct answer is going to increase dramatically from what you can achieve with Dr. Google—or your doctor, for that matter. Your searches on the Internet will then take on a different form: you will not be asking what is the matter with you so much as asking what the best treatment is. For example, you'll be correlating your data with that of others with similar disorders via social media to see what works best. And you'll be bringing potential therapeutic options in addition to diagnostic information to your doctor, and conferring with him or her about the best way to treat the disease you have or the disorder you're trending towards.

The reason that diagnoses made by questioning the digital you will become so accurate is that the molecular-level information contained there is starting to provide many readily measured molecular biomarkers—in the form of genetic features or levels of particular proteins, for example—that give precise information about your risk of disease or your actual disease. Genetic biomarkers have long been used to diagnose inherited diseases, of which there are multitudes. One example concerns lipid-storage diseases such as Gaucher's disease, which is caused by a mutation in a protein called lysosomal glucocerebrosidase, which breaks down a class of relatively insoluble compounds known as sphingolipids. Gaucher's disease can be definitively diagnosed by detecting mutations in the gene coding for this protein. The consequences of Gaucher's disease are severe: the most aggressive form causes death by age two due to brain damage. These lipid-storage diseases are relatively rare, with an incidence of between 1 in 40,000 to 1 in 120,000 live births, and affect a few thousand people worldwide.[4] However, they are examples of genetic ailments that can be detected by a simple genetic biomarker. Prenatal screens for these biomarkers often result in a decision to abort.

An area known as pharmacogenomics, which concerns the relation between your genotype and the effects that drugs will have on you, provides another example of how early precursors to the complete digital you are influencing medical practice. Taking the wrong drug can have terrible consequences if you have the wrong genetic makeup for dealing with that drug. In addition, it would be good to know if the prescribed drug will actually work for you. The danger is compounded by the drug culture we live in. Fifty percent of North Americans take one prescribed drug or another, and people over sixty-five average five or more drugs, which leads to a high potential for adverse drug reactions.

The irony is that for many drugs, we already know the genetic markers that predict bad side effects. More than 120 drugs approved by the Federal Drug Administration (FDA) have known genetic biomarkers to guide whether a particular person should or should not take that drug.[5] These biomarkers are often stated on the package insert that accompanies the drug when you pick it up from the pharmacist. This information is, of course, currently completely useless, because neither you nor your doctor know what your genetic profile is and consequently whether you will react well or badly to any drug he or she prescribes. Drug prescription is therefore a trial-and-error process, and a rather dangerous one. The application of pharmacogenomics—correlating your genetic makeup to the way your body will deal with a particular drug—has the potential to fix all that. All you will have to do is ask your digital self what effect that drug will have on you.

Pharmacogenomics has been used to guide whether or not a drug should be prescribed for a particular individual for some time. But these tests are usually used one by one in a hospital setting to discover whether or not a particular drug will work. For instance, the anticancer drug Herceptin is used to treat breast cancer. If your cancer cells do not make the protein that Herceptin binds to, Herceptin will do nothing for you; therefore, a simple genetic test is often done to help doctors decide whether or not to use it.

The problem is that we need these tests to be generally available for more commonly used drugs, including drugs sold over the counter. Tylenol, or acetaminophen, is among the most widely used pain relievers and is considered a very safe drug. But for people with a mutation in a gene called CD44, Tylenol can cause acute liver injury; even the recommended dosages can be life threatening.[6] For other drugs, our genes determine the dose we should get. Warfarin is a blood thinner prescribed to heart attack and stroke patients to prevent blood clots. People who have a mutation in a gene called *VKORC1*—which corresponds to roughly 37 percent of Caucasians and 14 percent of people of African descent—metabolize Warfarin poorly and so should receive a smaller dose of the drug to minimize adverse effects.[7] Ninety percent of commonly prescribed drugs are broken down in your liver by proteins belonging to the cytochrome P450 (CYP) family.[8] The dose an individual receives should be adjusted depending on whether a person over-expresses or under-expresses the proteins that break down the drug; otherwise, the drug may not work or may produce unacceptable toxicity.

The need to make these genetic tests available to all of us to protect us from adverse drug reactions is obvious—especially given the multitude of drugs being prescribed for us. And it's beginning to happen. In Indiana, for example, David Flockhart is introducing a simple genetic test to guide prescription practices in a hospital outpatient setting for approximately fifty commonly prescribed drugs, with the aim of improving outcomes and preventing adverse drug reactions.[9] Similarly, Martin Dawes is leading efforts in British Columbia to introduce a genetic test to guide prescription practices by family doctors for more than 100 drugs.[10] This testing targets patients who are over sixty-five and who are taking ten or more drugs— a population that is at high risk for adverse drug reactions. Remarkably, this innovation marks the first time in the world that family doctors, who write 85 percent of drug prescriptions in North America, will have access to genetic information to help them make more informed decisions—despite the fact that in many cases, the genetic information to influence drug prescription has been available for twenty years or more.

A central focus of the work of Flockhart and Dawes is the development of clinical decision support systems (CDSS) to assist physicians in interpreting the genetic data. Although all physicians know that genetic differences can influence a patient's response to a drug, very few have received formal training in pharmacogenomics. The CDSS will be computer-based and will first be generated by an expert panel consisting of physicians with extensive experience in pharmacogenomics and genetic counseling. Once the panel reaches consensus regarding recommended prescription practices for a patient with a given set of genetic biomarkers, a computer algorithm will be written that will reach the same decisions as the expert panel. This algorithm will be programmed into the patient's EMR so that when a doctor types in a drug prescription for a patient, a pop-up will appear to indicate whether that drug is suited to that patient and what an appropriate dose would be. The assistance given by the CDSS is the thin edge of the wedge. Such support systems will become more sophisticated and more predictive as more data, including whole-genome sequences or other proteome and microbiome data, are added to the digital version of you.

The need for pharmacogenomic tests to guide individualized administration of anticancer drugs is even more acute and is only slowly being addressed. Here, your digital self in the form of your genome can be used to determine whether or not you'll have a bad side effect from a chemotherapy drug. A Canadian trial group is playing a leading role here to prevent adverse drug reactions in children. The group, called the Genotype-Specific Approaches to Therapies in Childhood (GATC), is led by Michael Hayden and Bruce Carleton and is focused on cisplatin-induced deafness and doxorubicin-induced cardiotoxicity (heart toxicity).[11] Cisplatin is an extremely important and effective drug for the treatment of cancer. More than one million new patients are dosed with cisplatin every year for treatment of liver, ovarian, brain, lung, bladder, and head and neck cancers. However, cisplatin is also a very nasty drug. Among other side effects, it causes permanent hearing loss in 10 percent to 38 percent of patients. The situation is even worse for children under fourteen: nearly 40 percent will develop severe hearing loss.

Why do some children develop severe hearing loss while others don't? Is it related to their genetic makeup? Hayden and Carleton are addressing those questions. They recruited more than 160 children and compared the genotype of children who went deaf as a result of treatment with cisplatin with the genotype of children who did not. They found that for children with mutations in a gene associated with hearing called COMT (catechol-O-methyltransferase), there was a 90 percent chance of deafness if they were treated with cisplatin.[12] Some children who did not have that mutation still went deaf when treated with cisplatin. Now the hunt is on for other genes involved in hearing that might also be affected by cisplatin, which will improve the sensitivity of the test.

Well, you may say, that is all very well, but is there a drug that could be substituted for cisplatin if the child tested positive for potential hearing loss, and wouldn't you be putting the child's life in jeopardy if you didn't use cisplatin? This is true, but the genetic test spurs research into drugs that protect against the toxic effects of cisplatin. Other research is aimed at developing ways to deliver cisplatin more specifically to the tumor while avoiding tissues that play a role in hearing. The presence of the genetic test as a "companion diagnostic" provides an incentive for developing such drugs. Companies that make these drugs will be able to identify the patients who will benefit and will be able to charge a premium for their product.

Genetic testing for the risk of a toxic side effect such as hearing loss can have unexpected emotional consequences. A pediatric physician tells a story of a patient of his, a three-year-old girl, who had brain cancer. Her prognosis was bad: the doctor estimated she had perhaps six months to live, possibly nine months if chemotherapy were used. The parents asked if she could be tested for susceptibility to hearing loss before they agreed to chemotherapy that included cisplatin. The doctor asked, "Why? You'll gain a bit more time with your child if we treat her, whether or not she tests positive." The father responded, "Doctor, you don't understand. My daughter has just begun to talk; in fact, she can speak two languages [the parents came from different ethnic backgrounds]. We want to be able to talk with her as long as we can."

Doxorubicin is another horrible cancer drug that is widely used to treat blood cancers, breast cancer, and most childhood cancers. Nearly a million people receive this drug every year in North America. It is highly effective: the improvement in childhood cancer survival rates from approximately 30 percent in the 1960s to greater than 80 percent today can be attributed in part to the use of doxorubicin. But it is still a horrible drug. Heart function can be significantly compromised in 10 percent to 30 percent of patients; in severe cases, heart failure can occur, resulting in a mortality rate of more than 60 percent. Approximately 20 percent of children receiving doxorubicin will have reduced heart function for life or will require a heart transplant. But the response of patients to doxorubicin is highly variable. Some patients can tolerate three times the normal dose, while others suffer heart damage at any dose. Again, by comparing the genetic profiles of people who can tolerate high doses of doxorubicin with those who cannot, researchers are beginning to uncover a biomarker to guide whether an individual should receive a low dose—or any dose at all—as part of a chemotherapy regime. The particular biomarker in this case is a mutation in a protein that pumps drugs such as doxorubicin out of cells. The test can predict, with 75 percent accuracy,[13] those who will suffer cardiotoxicity. Luckily, in this case, there is a potential substitute for those at risk: a formulation of doxorubicin packaged into small vesicles that has similar potency but has much-reduced cardiotoxic potential.

Biomarkers are being developed and validated for many other anticancer drugs to identify those at unacceptable risk. Examples include vincristine and drugs based on Taxol, which can produce peripheral nerve damage leading to numbness or pain in your hands and feet. But drugs that are very toxic, such as many anticancer drugs, are not the only ones with risks. Many commonly used drugs have major risks too. For example, there is a clear need to identify whether you rapidly metabolize painkillers such as codeine. Codeine works as a painkiller because it is metabolized in your body to produce morphine by a protein in your liver called CYP2D6. Some people have more than one copy of this gene or have other mutations that result in very rapid conversion of codeine to morphine.[14] So if you are a new mother who is a fast metabolizer, breastfeeding your child and using codeine to manage postpartum pain can lead to potentially lethal levels of morphine in your infant's bloodstream. You definitely need to know this information beforehand.

The identification of mutations in your genome is increasingly enabling the development of individualized therapies. A major example concerns monoclonal antibodies. Antibodies are proteins produced by your immune system to recognize invaders such as bacteria or viruses. Antibodies bind to specific molecules (termed antigens) on the surface of target cells such as bacteria, cancer cells, or cells infected by a virus and tag the cell for destruction by other components of the immune system. In the mid-1970s, César Milstein and colleagues at Cambridge University found ways of producing large amounts of monoclonal antibodies (MAbs) that could recognize almost any desired antigen on a cell surface.[15] This ability has led to the development of MAbs that recognize personalized, patient-specific antigens. The best known example is Herceptin, a MAb that binds to the HER-2 protein, which is over-expressed in approximately 25 percent of early-stage breast cancers and can lead to improved survival for patients suffering from metastatic breast cancer.[16] In this case, a genetic test is first performed to determine whether the patient's tumor is over-expressing the HER-2 protein, as Herceptin will have no benefit if it doesn't.

Other drugs are appearing that target specific disease-causing proteins made by defective genes that have been identified through genetic analyses. These molecularly targeted drugs very specifically inhibit the function of a particular protein associated with a disease. For instance, about 4 percent of patients with non-small-cell lung cancer have a mutation that drives cancer growth due to a protein that is the product of two genes fused together. A drug called Xalkori inhibits the defective gene product and can shrink or stabilize the tumors in most patients carrying the causative gene. Richard Heimler, a father of two and an active member of the Lung Cancer Alliance, was diagnosed with non-small-cell lung cancer at age forty-four. He writes[17]

> I had pneumonectomy [lung removal] surgery of my right lung in 2004. Two years later, I was diagnosed with a small malignant brain tumor that was removed surgically. This was followed with six months of chemotherapy. A year later, I was diagnosed with a small malignant tumor under my ribs and it was successfully removed. A year later, I was diagnosed with another small brain tumor and had gamma knife radiation to successful [sic] destroy the tumor. A year later, I was diagnosed with multiple small tumors on my left lung and immediately began chemotherapy.

After testing positive for the particular mutation Xalkori targets, Heimler was treated with the drug in an experimental trial. Today, he reports that his tumors no longer show up on CT scans, a testament to the potency of personalized therapies. Xalkori received FDA approval in late 2012.[18]

Kalydeco is another targeted drug used to treat a monogenic disease—that is, a disease caused by only one defective gene. Cystic fibrosis (CF) is a monogenic disease arising from defects in the CFTR gene that codes for the CFTR protein that transports chloride ions across cell membranes. Patients with CF have thick, sticky mucus in the lungs that causes chronic lung infections; other symptoms include scarring of the pancreas, impaired digestion, and infertility. As recently as the 1980s, people with CF didn't live much longer than fourteen years, but today they have a life expectancy of approximately thirty-five years primarily because of improvements in managing the disease, such as ways of dislodging the mucus in the lungs.[19] Kalydeco, however, is aimed at curing the disease rather than managing it. The drug binds to a version of a defective CFTR protein that is found in 3 percent to 5 percent of people with CF and improves its ability to function.[20] Alex Parker of Victoria, Australia, was diagnosed with CF when she was six months old and lived with the condition for twenty-three years before a genetic analysis showed that she carried the particular mutation that Kalydeco could treat. Parker describes CF as producing the congestion and lethargy of a bad cold, along with bloating and a stomachache:[21]

You wake up every morning struggling to breathe. You feel nauseous after you eat. You force yourself to exercise in hope that it might just move the mucus from your lungs. Then one day they give you two little blue pills a day and all your suffering almost instantly stops. Your dreams start to become a reality and you start living a normal, energetic and fun-filled life. This is what happened to me. This is what happened to me the moment I started on Kalydeco.

Another testament to treatment based on a highly personalized approach, for sure.

Genetic biomarkers are also leading to dramatic measures to prevent disease. The BRCA1 gene is expressed in breast tissue and in the ovaries, and codes for a protein that either helps repair damaged (mutated) DNA or triggers a suicide process to destroy the cell if repair is not possible. A mutation in the BRCA1 gene can lead to a defective repair or cell suicide protein, allowing the cells to proliferate unchecked. Women who carry that mutation have about a 60 percent chance of developing breast cancer in their lifetime (versus 12 percent in the general population), and a 40 percent chance of developing ovarian cancer.[22]

Mutations in the BRCA1 gene therefore provide an important biomarker for the risk of developing breast cancer. Knowing whether or not you have that biomarker can have considerable impact, as illustrated by the case of the actress Angelina Jolie. Her mother died from breast cancer at age fifty-six. Jolie had her genome analyzed at age thirty-eight and found that she was positive for the BRCA1 mutation. According to Jolie, doctors told her that her risk of developing breast cancer with her particular mutation was 87 percent. In 2013, she acted preemptively, undergoing a double mastectomy. She wrote, "Cancer is a word that strikes fear into people's hearts, producing a deep sense of powerlessness. But today it is possible to find out through a blood test whether you are highly susceptible to breast and ovarian cancer, and then take action." She continued, "The decision to have a mastectomy was not easy. But it is one I am very happy that I made. My chances of developing breast cancer have dropped from 87 percent to under 5 percent. I can tell my children that they don't need to fear they will lose mc to breast cancer."[23]

Genetic analyses can also be used to develop personalized therapies aimed at infectious diseases such as HIV/AIDS. As is well known, viruses mutate rapidly, and the strain that one patient is infected with may well differ from the strain infecting another patient. Julio Montaner, director of the British Columbia Centre for Excellence in HIV/AIDS, is using genetic analyses to detect the particular genetic profile of the virus a patient is infected with. As he says, "This technology will be invaluable to the lives of our patients. We will be able to quickly treat patients by delivering personalized medicine based on their unique strain of the virus. This will help us save time and money while also significantly decreasing the number of new HIV and AIDS cases."[24] For Montaner, this represents the next step in his long battle against HIV/AIDS. He was a major contributor to the introduction of anti-HIV triple drug therapies in the 1990s that effectively changed HIV/AIDS from a lethal disease to a chronic condition.

Genetic biomarkers for hereditary diseases also help to focus efforts to treat diseases where preventive efforts are not possible. In 1993, researchers identified a link between a gene called *ApoE*, which codes for a protein involved in transporting cholesterol in your blood and in your brain, and late-onset Alzheimer's disease. *ApoE* has three variants known as *ApoE2*, *ApoE3*, and *ApoE4*. Individuals who carry two copies of the *ApoE4* gene have twenty times the risk of developing Alzheimer's disease compared with the general population.[25] This finding has focused research on the relationship between *ApoE4* and Alzheimer's disease, including determining whether or not *ApoE* has a role in dissolving the distinctive amyloid plaques associated with Alzheimer's disease.

The discovery of biomarkers such as the *ApoE4* gene also poses a dilemma for those who may be at high risk for currently incurable diseases such as Alzheimer's or Huntington's disease. The question is, if there is no cure, do you want to know that you're going to get it? Overall, anecdotal evidence suggests about half the population will adopt a passive approach and either will not want to be tested for inherited diseases or, if they are, will want to have information given to them only for actionable disorders—disorders for which there is a treatment. The other half will want to know the data in its entirety and act on it to try to reduce their risks.

And, in the end, it is important to know what your risks are, because there are always things that you can do, some of which are not intuitively obvious. Researchers at the University of British Columbia in Vancouver recently performed a study on women aged seventy to eighty with mild cognitive impairment.[26] These women were assigned to one of three groups: weight training, aerobic training, or balance-and-tone training. In each program, participants exercised two times a week for six months. At the end of the study, those who had participated in weight training fared best: they outperformed the other groups on tests measuring attention, memory, and higher-order brain functions like conflict resolution.

So weight lifting might help prevent or delay dementia. Who'd have thought? When you think about it, though, maybe it makes sense. When you're exercising, particularly when you're lifting a heavy weight, you're not just exercising the muscle that is lifting the weight; you are also exercising the nerve that is sending the message to the muscle to lift the weight. These nerves are hard-wired into your brain, and the more you strain your muscles, the harder your nerves fire to stimulate the muscle. Nerves consist of bundles of neurons, the same cell types that are also involved in higher brain processes such as perception and consciousness. In the same way that exercise has been shown to stimulate production of stem cells in muscle, it is possible that by exercising your nerves, you induce more neuron stem cells in your brain. Which is presumably a good thing for cognitive function.

Other good things can come from knowing about a genetic problem you might have, even if there is no treatment. As detailed in Elaine Westwick's blog in 2011,[27] Angela Francesco's mother, and her grandmother, had Huntington's disease, a degenerative condition affecting muscle coordination and cognition, inexorably leading to death. Huntington's is caused by a mutation of the Huntington gene—the *HTT* gene—and unlike the *BRCA* or *ApoE* genes, where having the mutation only increases your risk for disease, the *HTT* mutation guarantees it. Francesco hadn't wanted to know her own status—until she made marriage plans. She got tested for the Huntington's genetic biomarker, and the news was not good: "When we walked out of the clinic, I was devastated. I just could not imagine how life would continue. But it did. I was back at work the next day, we started planning our future, a big holiday, our wedding, our house together, our plans for children . . ." Her desire to have a child free of Huntington's drove her and her husband to use in vitro fertilization using a donor egg, and she became pregnant. On her blog, Francesco wrote, "Someone has given us an unbelievable gift, and with that we have stopped a fatal disease (in our family) for generations to come."

Genomic biomarkers are being used not only to predict adverse reactions to drugs but also to guide therapy. The major focus of personalized medicine as it is practiced today is identifying genetic biomarkers found in cancerous cells and using this information to guide cancer therapy. Massive efforts are underway to shift from the current system, in which patients are treated according to where their cancer originates (breast, lung, prostate, pancreas, etc.), to a system in which the treatment is based, at least in part, on the genetic makeup of their cancer. This shift is enabled by the availability of ever-cheaper sequencing capabilities, but there are many challenges. Identifying the so-called driver mutations that are actually helping the cancer cell grow is a particular problem. These are the ones you want to interfere with. And then there's the issue of finding drugs that inhibit expression of the driver genes or interfere with the function of the proteins they produce.

The scale of the efforts that are being made to improve cancer therapy using genetically based personalized approaches is truly impressive. The MD Anderson Cancer Center in Houston is conducting a $3 billion "moonshot" program to cure breast, leukemia, lung, and prostate cancer using protocols based on gene-sequencing technology.[28] Genomics England has announced a program to sequence the genomes of up to 100,000 cancer patients and the genomes of their cancers.[29] The Ontario Institute for Cancer Research has instituted a billion-dollar program to "cure cancer in our lifetime" using personalized medicine approaches with an emphasis on cancer-genome sequencing. There is not a major cancer center in Europe or North America that does not have a large-scale initiative with similar intentions. Is it working? Stories are beginning to emerge that give rise to optimism.

The first example of how genomic data can influence cancer treatment was reported in the journal *Genome Biology* in 2010 by researchers at the BC Cancer Agency in Vancouver and concerned a patient who presented with a cancer on his tongue.[30] The first stage of treatment was to surgically remove the tumor, followed by irradiation to kill any cancer cells that were missed. The irradiation didn't work or was too late; subsequently, the patient developed lung cancer as a result of metastases that had traveled to his lung. Biopsies were then taken of the tumor tissue in the lung, and these were subjected to genome sequencing. It was found that a gene called receptor tyrosine kinase (*RET*), which is known to promote cancer growth, was expressed thirty-five times more in the tumor tissue than in normal tissues. A drug called sunitinib was identified that inhibits function of the *RET* protein; when this was administered, the lung tumors shrank significantly, and the disease remained stable for five months. After that, however, the tumors started to grow again. Genome sequencing of the tumors revealed that new mutations had appeared. Unfortunately, no drugs could be identified to disable the proteins made by these defective genes, and the patient died. Nonetheless, without the genetic analysis, sunitinib would not have been used to treat this patient, and the initial response would not have been observed, illustrating the importance of genetic information for identifying the drugs that will work on any particular cancer.

The story of Lukas Wartman is another example. As described in a *New York Times* article published in 2012,[31] Wartman developed acute lymphoblastic leukemia (ALL), a devastating disease that has a five-year survival rate of 40 percent. For individuals who relapse after initial chemotherapy, as was the case for Wartman, the survival rate drops to 10 percent.

Analysis of Wartman's DNA and RNA by researchers at Washington University indicated that his leukemic cells were making large amounts of a protein called FLT3, and this protein could be a driver of cell division. Interestingly, sunitinib also inhibits FLT3. When this drug was administered to Wartman, his cancer promptly went into remission, allowing Wartman to undergo a potentially curative stem cell transplant. The genetic information was vital because sunitinib is not usually used to treat ALL. Without the genetic analysis, Wartman's doctors would not have thought of using it. So there is reason to hope that one day you will have cancer drugs that actually work on the type of cancer you have, as opposed to the current situation in which there is only a 25 percent chance they will be effective.

For diseases other than cancer and inherited diseases, biomarkers based on genetic data only provide information on your risk of disease but do not tell you whether you actually have that disease. However, biomarkers based on your protein profiles in body fluids such as blood, saliva, or urine will tell you what disorder you actually have. We have had blood tests to detect proteins that are biomarkers for disease for many years, but most of these measure single proteins (or metabolites) such as C-reactive protein to diagnose inflammation, alkaline phosphatase to ascertain liver damage, creatinine to detect kidney damage, glucose to determine sugar levels, or troponin 1 to detect damage from a heart attack. Your blood, however, contains a tremendous amount of additional information that we haven't yet tapped.

Cancers also secrete proteins into your blood in the same way that proteins from your heart, liver, lungs, and kidneys are secreted into the circulation, providing potential blood tests for cancer. For example, lung cancer is the leading cause of cancer death (3 million cases every year in the U.S.), and the lung nodules that may be cancerous are usually visualized by CT scans as lesions of various sizes. Small lesions less than 0.9 centimeters in diameter are treated by "watchful waiting" to see if they will grow—growth being a sign of malignancy. Large lesions bigger than 2 centimeters in diameter are treated by surgery, leaving approximately 600,000 people, whose nodules measure 0.9 to 2 centimeters, in a "dilemma zone," where diagnoses of cancer are attempted by using positron emission tomography (PET) scans or biopsies. Biopsies are invasive and can be dangerous to your health, both procedures are very costly, and the combined results are often not definitive. A Seattle-based company called Integrated Diagnostics has developed a blood test that measures the levels of 13 proteins in the blood (selected from an initial panel of 400) and can tell whether a lung nodule is benign with 90 percent accuracy, thereby accounting for approximately 70 percent of nodules in the dilemma zone.[32] The test clearly offers peace of mind for a considerable number of patients, and in addition, it has the potential to save the U.S. health-care system approximately $3.5 billion annually by preventing unnecessary PET scans and biopsies. Similar molecular-level blood tests can be expected to become available for many forms of cancer and will become more accurate as time goes on.

A precise knowledge of the proteins associated with disease is also giving rise to entirely new classes of drugs based on gene therapy. For those who are not familiar with how new drugs are developed, the usual process is haphazard, slow, and extremely expensive. Typically, a protein is identified that may be involved in some disease process, such as a protein that drives cancer growth. Then attempts are made to find "small molecules" that can stop that protein from functioning. All the drugs that are familiar to you, that you take every day to cure a headache or arthritic pain or an infection, such as aspirin or ibuprofen or penicillin, are molecules that are small enough to be able to get inside cells to reach the proteins they interact with.

Finding the right small molecule for a new target protein can involve screening hundreds of thousands of small molecules to find one that interacts with the protein and inhibits its function. Then an interminable amount of time is spent using chemistry to try to make the molecule better—more potent and more amenable to administration either orally or by injection. Following that, detailed animal studies are required to show that the molecule actually works to cure the target disease and is not so toxic that it kills the animals. These studies are followed by hugely expensive and time-consuming clinical trials—first to find a safe dose in people (Phase I), then to find if the drug can cure the target disease in people (Phase II), and then to compare it to the best available therapy currently used to treat the disease (Phase III). Only then is there a possibility that the drug will be approved by regulatory agencies such as the FDA. This process takes on average fifteen years and can cost a billion dollars if the cost of drugs that fail to make the grade are included. And at the end of it, you have a drug that goes everywhere in the body, not just where you need it, and that can be guaranteed to have a nasty side effect on some portion of the population in some region of their bodies.

There must be a better way to develop new drugs that work for you, and there are reasons for optimism. This is due to improved molecular-level understanding of the disease and underlying biology. For example, the genetic disease called familial hypercholesterolemia leads to high levels of low-density lipoprotein (LDL) in the blood, the so-called "bad" cholesterol. LDL contains a protein called ApoB100, leading to the possibility that if we could inhibit production of ApoB100 in a targeted way, we could reduce LDL levels. Once you have decided what your target protein is, you immediately know the sequence of the gene in the genome that codes for that protein, because the sequence of amino acids in the protein is determined by the sequence of bases in the gene. In turn, knowing the gene sequence allows for a precise way to develop new drugs based on DNA or RNA that inhibit production of the target protein. If you introduce a short (approximately twenty base pairs is usual) piece of DNA (an oligomer) into a cell, it will bind specifically to a region of the genomic DNA with a sequence complementary to the oligomer and prevent the gene that contains that sequence from being expressed. Therefore, the protein the gene codes for will no longer be made. This process is often referred to as "gene silencing." Complementary means that the C, T, A, G on the oligomer line up with their complementary bases G, A, T, C on the genomic DNA. The short pieces of DNA, known as antisense molecules, can be developed quickly compared to small-molecule drugs and can potentially be used to treat a wide range of diseases. Kynamro, the first systemic antisense drug to gain FDA approval in January 2013,[33] inhibits production of ApoB100 and significantly reduces LDL levels in the blood. Clinical trials are in progress for other antisense treatments for disorders ranging from inflammatory diseases to blood clotting disorders, to Duchenne's muscular dystrophy, a rare genetic musculoskeletal disease.

Short sequences of RNA that bind to mRNA coding for the target protein can be used in a similar fashion. The advantage of the RNA approach is that it is catalytic: the presence of one piece of RNA can lead to the destruction of many mRNAs that contain a complementary sequence. The RNA molecules used to bind to the mRNA and cause its destruction are called short interfering RNA (siRNA) and again can be made quickly once you know the protein that you wish to "silence." siRNA can potentially be used to treat all the diseases that antisense drugs can, but with greater potency. The Ebola virus, for example, is a contagious hemorrhagic virus that can lead to bleeding internally and through the nose, mouth, and other bodily orifices. It kills approximately 70 percent of people infected. The Ebola virus, like other viruses, is taken up into cells in your body, where it takes over cellular machinery to make more copies of itself. These new copies of the virus then go on to infect other cells. A collaboration between a Vancouver-based company, Tekmira Pharmaceuticals, and the U.S. Department of Defense has shown that intravenous delivery of siRNA that silences the genes Ebola requires to replicate can result in 100 percent cures for animals infected with the virus.[34]

The antisense or siRNA approach has the potential for another benefit: the development of personalized drugs. For instance, as cancer progresses, many mutations can creep into the genome of the cancer cells, with the result that each person's cancer becomes a rare disease, requiring individualized treatment. In some cases, drugs to inhibit the causal proteins will already exist; but in many cases, drugs to affect these proteins will not be available. However, siRNA molecules, that will very effectively silence the offending proteins if they can be delivered to the tumor cells, can be made within a week or so. Thus one can envisage a rapid interplay between identification of new target proteins as the tumor produces new mutations, and the development of new siRNA medicines to control and reverse the tumor growth that results. It is likely that such medicines will be tested in humanized mouse "avatars," in which your tumor is grown and the effects of the siRNA medicine are monitored to see if it is effective before it is administered to you.

An area of explosive growth of personalized therapies for cancer involves finding ways to activate the immune system to fight cancer. That such an approach is possible stems from an observation by a physician named William Coley in the 1890s. Coley noted a patient who had a terminal form of cancer who contracted a severe bacterial infection. After the patient recovered from the infection, his cancer regressed, indicating that the infection somehow activated the patient's immune system to fight the cancer as well as the infection. In the 1950s Lewis Thomas and Frank Macfarlane Burnet suggested that the immune system could eradicate tumors by recognizing specific molecules on the surface of the tumor cells, and that cancers that progress somehow evade this immune surveillance.[35] These observations have stimulated considerable research, now coming to fruition, on how cancer cells evade detection and elimination by the immune system.

Most of this progress is due to an improved understanding of how the immune system works. Briefly, the key players are dendritic cells (DCs), T cells, and natural killer (NK) cells. DCs can be thought of as the generals of the immune system: they direct the production of "soldiers" in the form of T cells and NK cells, which are targeted to kill infected cells or cancer cells. However, to cause the targeted T cells and NK cells to be made, the DCs must first identify the infected cell or the cancer cell and then go through a maturation process. If the cancer cell is able to avoid detection or prevent the DCs from maturing, then the cancer will continue to grow. To bypass this problem, scientists are developing ways to take T cells or NK cells from the patient, engineer them so that they recognize the cancer cells, and then infuse them back into the patient. A very personalized approach!

The T cell method is showing remarkable results. First T cells are isolated from a patient's blood, and then a virus is used to insert a gene coding for a receptor on the surface of the T cell that recognizes cancer cells. These genetically modified T cells are then mass produced and infused back into the patient. As reported at the American Society of Hematology meeting in December 2013, incredible results have been achieved in initial trials in children suffering from leukemia caused by uncontrolled growth of B cells, the cells that produce antibodies.[36] B cells have a protein on their surface known as CD19. When T cells were made that express a receptor for CD19, and then given to the patients, nineteen of twenty-two children experienced complete responses. Some of these children had gone through more than ten previous therapies without success. "Our results demonstrate the potential of this treatment for patients who truly have no other therapeutic option," Dr. Stephan Grupp of the University of Pennsylvania said. "In the relatively short time that we've observed these patients, we have reason to believe that this treatment could become a viable therapy for their relapsed, treatment-resistant disease." Similar spectacular results have been observed in adults who showed complete responses in fourteen of sixteen cases. In some patients, up to seven pounds of tumor were eliminated in just a few weeks.

As with any therapy, there are downsides. A kidney problem known as tumor lysis syndrome can result from an overload of dead and dying tumor cells. Elevated levels of immunostimulatory molecules in the circulation can also cause problems but these can be controlled through the use of immunosuppressive drugs. A major concern is how this exquisitely personalized therapy, which requires sophisticated facilities for T cell isolation and genetic engineering, can be extended to thousands of patients. There is also the question of whether or not this approach can be translated into the treatment of solid tumors, which often have more effective tactics to avoid detection by the immune system. However, the point has been made: appropriate stimulation of the immune system can cure cancer.

The advent of the personalized medicine revolution has been accompanied by many ethical and societal issues. An early example is Louise Brown, who was conceived by in vitro fertilization in 1978: the world's first "test-tube" baby. Although her birth was a major medical achievement that offered infertile couples hope for their own biological children, it also raised a host of ethical concerns. The issues, which ranged from the appropriateness of surrogate mothers to the legal status of fertilized eggs, have still not been resolved and are set to become even more complicated. In 2013, the U.K. became the first country in the world to announce plans allowing "three-parent children."[87] The process by which a three-parent child could come into being potentially addresses diseases such as Kearns–Sayre syndrome, a condition characterized by weakness or paralysis of eye muscles and by abnormalities in heart function. Kearns-Sayre syndrome is caused by mutations in the DNA in the mitochondria—the power plants of the cell. Mitochondria—and therefore their DNA—are passed down from mother to child, through the egg, not through the nuclear DNA, which is a combination of the DNA from the mother and father. The idea of three-parent children is that an embryo's nuclear DNA—inherited from its mother and father—would be implanted in a donor egg with functional mitochondria. The child would have his or her parents' genetic material but would be spared the devastating effects of the defective mitochondria.

Other ethical issues concern the general availability of genetic information. Researchers need both healthy and unhealthy research participants to help answer the many important questions about the correlation between genotype and phenotype. Dan Roden, head of Vanderbilt University's personalized medicine program, has pointed out that "large numbers of patients, of diverse ancestries, are required to develop evidence to 'personalize' medicine."[38] In other words, to understand most genetic disorders, researchers have to sequence the DNA of hundreds of people with those disorders and then compare their DNA with that of thousands of people who do not have the disorder to get a statistically significant result that lets them determine the location and sequence of the faulty gene or genes. So do we have a moral duty to make our genes available for research?

Questions arise such as whether or not patients undergoing genetic testing should be told about incidental findings—like a potentially harmful mutation that researchers stumble across while looking for something else, or the fact that a patient's father isn't who he or she thinks he is. How much involvement should your family have in your decision to provide genetic information, given that information about your genes could also offer hints about theirs? Should researchers be allowed to use leftover samples from other studies for experimental purposes? The concerns are legion.

The issues being dealt with by legal, regulatory, and public policy groups as they try to deal with the consequences of molecular-level information about disease are another sign of the inroads molecular medicine is making. For example, can genes be patented? The *BRCA1* and *BRCA2* mutations that signify a high risk of breast cancer were patented by a company called Myriad Genetics, and as a result, the company had a stranglehold on the market. In a landmark case, Myriad's patents were challenged, and the case ended up in the Supreme Court in 2013. The judges handed down a unanimous decision that "a naturally occurring DNA segment is a product of nature and not patent eligible merely because it has been isolated."[39] This decision certainly favors progress: if patents were involved in the testing for each of the approximately 1,800 disease-associated genes discovered so far, the costs for testing for all of them would be out of reach for most people and for their insurers.

Regulatory agencies such as the FDA don't quite know what to do with biomarker tests that are, or are going to be, exceedingly accurate and that are sold directly to the consumer. Right now, the process for getting a biomarker test approved by the FDA as a diagnostic for a particular disease costs approximately $24 million USD. There are literally hundreds, if not thousands, of new diagnostics based on genomic, proteomic, and other molecular-level information that are making their way through clinical testing. Not all companies will want to go to the time and expense of achieving FDA certification, particularly if the market size for a specialized test does not warrant the expense. Such a test may be sold in regions such as the European Union, where the approval process is cheaper and faster. Alternatively companies could avoid making any precise diagnostic claims for their test but recommend you see your doctor if there is a problem. It won't take much detective work, however, to find out what they imply.

An early example concerns the experience of 23andMe, a company that, until recently, for $100, would provide you with a genetic profile indicating your risk for various diseases if you provided them with a vial of your saliva. In late 2013, the FDA issued a strong warning to 23andMe, which markets directly to consumers, saying:[40]

Some of the uses for which 23andMe's personal genome service is intended are particularly concerning, such as assessments for *BRCA*-related genetic risk and drug responses because of the potential health consequences that could result from false positive or false negative assessments for high-risk indications such as these. Assessments for drug responses carry the risks that patients relying on such tests may begin to self-manage their treatments through dose changes or even abandon certain therapies depending on the outcome of the assessment. For example, false genotype results for your warfarin drug response test could have significant unreasonable risk of illness, injury, or death to the patient due to thrombosis or bleeding events that occur from treatment with a drug at a dose that does not provide the appropriately calibrated anticoagulant effect.

In response to the FDA warning, 23andMe has stopped issuing health reports to new customers, offering only ancestry reports and raw genetic data. But we certainly haven't seen the end of the story. The calls from consumers and patients for diagnostic tests based on genetic, proteomic, metabolomic, microbiomic, and other biological data are becoming incredibly intense as these tests become ever more available and more accurate. There are now many companies that will give you not only genomic data but proteomic, metabolomic, and microbiomic information derived from a sample of your blood or fecal material that has considerable diagnostic content. You will want this information to help you diagnose disease or, as we shall see, to maintain wellness. How these pressures are handled will test the limits of the power of regulatory bodies around the world.

Regulatory bodies face other pressures resulting from an individualized approach to medicine. Personalized approaches are not very compatible with current drug testing and approval processes. A drug deemed unsafe in a classic clinical trial may, in fact, be safe—and effective—for patients with a particular genetic profile. Similarly, a drug considered ineffective for a majority of the population could be extremely effective for a small group of people with a particular genetic defect. Development of the beta-blocker drug bucindolol (Gencaro) was halted when a 2001 study showed that it didn't improve survival in patients with heart failure. But after the discovery that patients with two genetic variants that regulate heart function respond well to Gencaro, interest in the drug was rekindled, and new clinical trials—focused on those who have the genetic variants—are under way.[41] By coupling drug trials with genetic testing, researchers are able to more easily determine who will benefit from a drug and who will suffer adverse effects.

Regulatory issues also arise as we understand more about the biology of complicated diseases such as cancer. Molecular-level characterizations of these diseases reveal differences between the disease one person has as compared to another. As a result, more and more supposedly common diseases are becoming rare diseases. For example, advanced lung cancer can have eighty or more mutations; and a particular pattern of these mutations may be observed in only one patient. It is difficult to run a randomized, controlled trial, which regulatory agencies usually require for drug approval, when you have only one patient in it. The approach being developed here involves so-called n-of-1 clinical trials, in which the trial consists of the case study of a single person. Talk about personalized medicine! In n-of-1 trials, the sole participant would receive both the active drug and the placebo, and the randomization would be in the order of administration of test drugs. Although n-of-1 trials have been dismissed as providing merely anecdotal evidence, Nicholas Schork and his team at Scripps Health have made a compelling argument that "the ultimate goal of an n-of-1 trial is to determine the optimal or best intervention for an individual patient using objective data-driven criteria" and hence is "compatible with the ultimate end point of clinical practice: the care of individual patients."[42] For example, there are four major classes of antihypertensive drugs, and some physicians have used crossover rotations of these drugs to see which ones work best in individual patients, to the considerable benefit of the patient.

Societal issues arising from the practice of personalized medicine are proving to be just as contentious as the ethical concerns, if not more so. Prenatal genetic screening to identify children with Down's syndrome or Tay-Sachs disease or a myriad of other inherited genetic diseases is changing our societies in basic ways because most of these children are aborted. The introduction of a simple prenatal blood test to detect whether a child has Down's syndrome has resulted in a remarkable increase in abortions—more than 90 percent of such children are aborted in Europe, and only slightly less in North America,[43] leading to the possibility that in a generation or two, Down's syndrome may disappear, even though women are having children at a later age, which increases the chances of children being born with Down's syndrome. In addition, blood tests can now reveal many other things about an unborn child, including the sex. As a result, societies that do not value women are beginning to develop disruptive gender imbalances: for example, China will have nearly 40 million more men than women in 2020.[44] History suggests that such imbalances can be very destabilizing to societies.

This chapter has covered a lot of ground, and the message is clear. The impact of personalized, molecularly based medicine is already profound and increasing rapidly. The first versions of the digital you are being developed that include genetic information in addition to standard clinical data, and this information is being used to detect, diagnose, and guide treatment for genetic diseases ranging from inherited disorders to cancer, as well as to determine which drugs you should take and which you should avoid. Similarly, the digital version of you will soon be augmented by proteomic analyses of your blood to detect any disease you may have or may be trending towards, or whether the drugs you are taking or the lifestyle changes you are making are actually working. Drugs are being developed that are very specifically targeted to a particular disease you may have. And society is beginning to wrestle with the advent of technologies that tell you, with increasing accuracy, all about yourself. The groundwork for personalized medicine is in place and, for those in the vanguard, the revolution has begun.

6
PERSONALIZED MEDICINE IN THE NEXT TEN YEARS

WHAT MAJOR ADVANCES can we expect in the next ten years? As Yogi Berra said in his unique way, "Predictions are difficult, particularly about the future." But some things are clear. Personalized medicine is here to stay. It is going to spread as people acquire and share their digital data; it is going to become more accurate as big data analyses and technological advances lead to further improvements in our understanding of disease; it is going to be expanded into maintaining health in addition to identifying and treating disease; it is going to democratize medical care in the sense that very sophisticated diagnostics will become generally available to consumers; it is going to lead to enormous new industries aimed at maintaining wellness and treating potential rather than actual disease; it is going to completely disrupt current medical practices; and it is going to pose considerable ethical and social dilemmas. Many of these changes will arise from four areas where research activity is particularly intense: advances in gene therapy, improved understanding of brain function, investigations into the biology of aging, and the use of molecular-level medicine to maintain wellness.

Personalized medicine and gene therapy go hand in hand. The idea behind gene therapy is that if we can detect the genetic basis of a disease, that disease can be treated by inserting new genes into your genome in place of defective ones. The reasoning is straightforward: if a gene in your genome contains a mutation, leading to a protein that doesn't work properly, why not insert a functional copy of the gene into the genome? Putting this idea into practice has been somewhat difficult, however. For obvious reasons, your body has evolved elaborate defense mechanisms to prevent any invader from injecting its DNA or RNA into your genome.

Given that evolution has produced viruses that can insert their genome into the genome of target cells as part of the infective process, scientists have made great efforts to use viruses to replace defective genes in cells with functional versions. First attempts used modified viruses, containing the therapeutic gene, which could not be infective (that is, the virus could not replicate itself). However, the virus inserted the new gene into the genome of the target cell at random locations. This development proved risky because random insertion of DNA into your genome can potentially perturb expression of other genes and lead to new problems. Something like this process seems to have happened in gene-therapy trials in the early 2000s to treat children suffering from an immune disorder called X-linked severe combined immunodeficiency (X-SCID). X-SCID is often referred to as "bubble boy" disease because children suffering from this disease are extremely susceptible to infection, sometimes requiring a sterile chamber environment to avoid bacteria or viruses. Sadly, some of the children who received gene therapy for X-SCID to replace the defective gene developed leukemia a few years later. Researchers believe the random insertion of the gene activated an oncogene—a gene that can cause cancer.[1]

Another problem is that your immune system is programmed to recognize invading viruses and eliminate them from your body and also to kill cells that become infected by a virus. These immune reactions can be so intense that they are sometimes lethal. As discussed in a *New York Times* article published in 1999, Jesse Gelsinger suffered from ornithine transcarbamylase (OTC) deficiency, a rare genetic disorder that results in a buildup of ammonia due to incomplete breakdown of proteins.[2] In Jesse's case, this was controlled with a low-protein diet and drugs—thirty-two pills a day. In a quest to correct his OTC deficiency, Jesse was injected with a modified cold virus that contained the gene for OTC. The subsequent immune response was so strong that Jesse suffered multiple organ failure and died four days later. That was a black day not only for Jesse but also for gene therapy. Further development was halted for almost ten years.

These and other failures have led to some cynicism about the future of gene therapy for treating hereditary diseases such as Gaucher's or Huntington's, or diseases such as cancer. Claims that effective gene therapies are just around the corner and will provide a new method of curing hitherto incurable diseases are often dismissed as hyperbole. When an early version of the human genome sequence was announced in June 2000, Bill Clinton stated, "Genome science will revolutionize the diagnosis, prevention and treatment of most, if not all, human diseases. In coming years, doctors increasingly will be able to cure diseases like Alzheimer's, Parkinson's, diabetes and cancer by attacking their genetic roots... In fact, it is now conceivable that our children's children will know the term *cancer* only as a constellation of stars."[3] It hasn't quite turned out that way—yet. But there are signs of progress.

So what's changing now? The first gene-therapy drug was approved for human use by the European Medicines Agency in 2012: Glybera,[4] a drug to treat lipoprotein lipase (LPL) deficiency, a very rare (one in a million) inherited disease that can lead to severe pancreatitis. The delivery vehicle used is a virus that does not induce a strong immune response, known as adeno-associated virus (AAV), which is injected into the thigh muscle. The treatment has been shown to reduce lipid levels in the blood and prevent attacks of pancreatitis for up to two years. This success has led to other AAV-based gene therapies that are in development, including treatments for hemophilia, retinal degeneration, Parkinson's disease, and muscular dystrophy. Viruses are also proving useful for introducing genes into immune cells to enhance recognition of tumor cells, as discussed in the previous chapter.

As detailed in chapter 5, a form of gene therapy using antisense or siRNA oligonucleotides (short pieces of DNA or RNA, usually about twenty bases long) to silence target genes associated with disease is also increasingly successful. Isis Pharmaceuticals, a biotechnology company based in California, received FDA approval for Kynamro—a drug to treat high cholesterol by inhibiting production of a protein required to make LDL.[5] In addition, Alnylam Pharmaceuticals, a biotechnology company based in Boston, is developing a siRNA drug called patisiran which entered Phase III clinical trials in late 2013.[6] Patisiran silences a gene called transthyretin (*TTR*); mutations in the *TTR* gene cause defective TTR proteins to be made that can form insoluble amyloid plaques of denatured protein in heart and nerve tissue, causing heart failure and a progressive loss of sensation in the hands and feet. The only current treatment is a liver transplant. It is anticipated that the lower levels of TTR protein in the blood induced by patisiran will lead to reduced deposition of amyloid plaques, perhaps causing previously formed plaques to dissolve. There are many other DNA- or

RNA-based drugs in clinical development, and there is good reason to believe that they are going to be very effective.

So the future of gene therapy is increasingly bright. A particularly exciting development is that technology for manipulating your DNA is evolving rapidly. Nanosurgery on your DNA to correct defects may soon be an option. So-called CRISPR (clustered regularly interspersed short palindromic repeats) technology can be used to cut out the DNA of defective genes and insert the correct sequence. As Feng Zhang, a professor at MIT says, "We can go into the native genome, the natural DNA in the cell, and then make a modification in the genome to correct deleterious mutations."[7] This is incredible. Already this technique has been used to cure mice of genetic defects leading to cataracts and to insert DNA into the genome of stem cells to correct the cystic fibrosis gene. Other researchers are using the technique to delete a gene known as *pcsk9*, which can dramatically lower cholesterol levels, potentially providing a "vaccine" against heart disease.[8] So gene therapy is experiencing a remarkable renaissance, and many personalized, precise, and safe gene medicines are marching their way towards everyday clinical use.

Personalized medicine and your brain: that's a big one. Let's start with dementia, forgetting who you are. It doesn't get more personal than that. Dementia is a disease of old age, and its incidence doubles roughly every five years after the age of sixty-five. The prevalence of dementia in late old age is extreme, rising from 12 percent at age eighty to 22 percent for men and 30 percent for women at age ninety.[9] So you might want to live for a long time, but you'd better hope there's a cure for Alzheimer's disease and other disorders that cause cognitive impairment by the time you pass eighty. (Hopefully, something better than weight lifting.) You'll also need to save a lot of money: in the U.S. in 2010, the cost for care of demented people was in the range of $200 billion, taking into account the cost of assisted living.[10] This is not cheap: twenty-four-hour care can easily cost $100,000 a year. Your children may love you, but if they are paying, they may think wistfully of the days, possibly mythological, when the Inuit could ship their infirm elders out to sea on the nearest ice floe.

How about personalized medicine and your mental health? According to the National Alliance on Mental Illness, nearly one in two people in the U.S. will suffer from depression, anxiety disorders,[11] or another mental health problem at some point in their life, and about one in seventeen currently has a serious mental illness. Costs due to mental illness run in excess of $100 billion per year in lost productivity; in addition, schools have to offer special education, the court system is saturated with people who have mental disorders, and mental health problems culminating in suicide are a leading cause of death in younger people.

And then we have all the other problems that are brain related: Huntington's, Parkinson's, epilepsy, schizophrenia, autism, meningitis, stroke, concussion, brain tumors—the list goes on and on. And we are really not very good at treating any of these conditions. So is personalized medicine going to do anything about it? This is a tough question to answer. So far, personalized medicine for the brain is limited to attempts to tailor antidepressants and other drugs used to treat mental problems to avoid adverse drug reactions. Overall the field is fundamentally limited by a lack of understanding of how the brain works. So the question becomes, are we going to see improvements in our understanding of how the brain operates over the next decade, which can then be expected to lead to individualized solutions? The answer to that is, "Probably."

The central problem here is relating the biology of the brain to behavior. Activity in various parts of the brain can be observed in response to various stimuli using techniques such as functional magnetic resonance imaging (fMRI). However, despite many advances, the spatial resolution is still relatively poor. Each pixel of the fMRI image corresponds to at least 100,000 neurons; the firing of individual neurons cannot be detected. But it is crucial to detect these individual events. The thoughts you have are likely due to "emergent behavior" resulting from the simultaneous firing of thousands of neurons in your head. The term emergent behavior, in this case, refers to behavior that cannot be predicted by analysis of any one neuron; it is many neurons interacting together that enable your brain to think, act, and dream. The potential for emergent behavior in the brain is huge. There are approximately 11 billion neurons in your brain, and each of these has on average 7,000 connections with other neurons. Neurons are connected to each other by synapses that transmit electrical signals from one neuron to the next, so there are approximately 100 trillion individual synapses that can be firing at any one time. In the language of omics, this is called your connectome. It is a daunting task to map the connectome and correlate thousands, tens of thousands, or even greater numbers of synapses firing at once with your ability to remember, feel, see, and talk.

But there are many wild and wonderful new technologies that are attempting to do just that. Currently in development are nano-size sensors to detect electrical impulses when implanted deep in the brain, techniques to image the brain according to the voltage across the neural membrane (which corresponds to nerve firing), as well as optogenetics—inserting genes into neurons that respond to light by causing ions to flow across neural membranes, thus turning neurons on or off.

The information-processing demands are huge. As Rafael Yuste and George Church indicate in an article in *Scientific American* in 2014,[12] imaging the activity of all the neurons in a mouse brain could generate 300 petabytes of data in an hour. Compare this to storing your genome, a mere 800 gigabytes— about 400,000 times less data. Moving to the human brain will require considerably more data generation, storage, and analysis. But just as it was impossible for Watson and Crick to imagine sequencing the whole human genome in 1954, it would be unwise for us to say this kind of imaging can't happen within the next ten years.

So we can see the day coming when, thanks to one imaging technique or another, rudimentary maps of the brain activity associated with our moods, behavior, and actions will be achieved. It is not hard to envision that this will lead to some very personalized therapies, be they for depression, addiction, schizophrenia, or a host of other disorders, by simply interfering with the activity pattern associated with extremes of mood and behavior. Equally, of course, it could go the other way, with customers paying to be induced into a constant state of orgasm or other forms of ecstatic pleasure. Whether or not such therapies or indulgences will be available in ten years is certainly arguable, but it is likely that we will start to see the outlines of how to get there.

What about aging and personalized medicine? A focus on the elderly and treating aging as a potentially preventable disease makes sense in a lot of ways: the elderly consume a disproportionate share of the health-care budget, in large part because of chronic conditions such as dementia, arthritis, diabetes, and cardiovascular disease, to say nothing of more acute diseases such as cancer. The costs are huge: people aged sixty-five and over made up around 13 percent of the

U.S. population in 2002, but they consumed 36 percent of total U.S. personal health-care expenses.[13] In Canada, the current number is closer to 44 percent.[14] These costs are only going to increase as baby boomers cross the sixty-five-year-old threshold. Some estimates suggest a doubling in costs for the elderly by 2030. Whatever the numbers, the situation is clearly not sustainable.

You are probably not used to thinking that aging could be seen as a disease, and for that matter, neither is the FDA. It doesn't acknowledge aging to be a treatable condition. And promoting that concept, with its connotations of seeking immortality, certainly puts you in some fairly flaky company. But research aimed at understanding and treating aging processes has gained respectability and has generated some credible approaches.

The telomere story, for example, is becoming increasingly persuasive. In the early 1960s, Leonard Hayflick, a professor at Stanford University, discovered that when human fetal cells were cultivated in a medium that contained all the essential ingredients to keep cells happy, they divided approximately fifty times, then stopped and entered a period of senescence. Senescence means that the cells became "old" and either committed suicide by a process called apoptosis or remained alive but exhibited different gene-expression profiles from their precursors, indicating altered, presumably reduced, functional capabilities. In the 1970s, it was discovered that the ends of the DNA strands in chromosomes contain regular repeats of DNA sequences, dubbed telomeres, and that when a cell divides, it does not completely replace these DNA repeats; in other words, the telomere gets shorter every time a cell divides. This finding was finally used to explain the "Hayflick limit": if the telomeres become short enough, then the cells can no longer divide.

As a result, the study of telomeres has become a central feature of aging research because it suggests that the reason you get old and die is because your telomeres get shorter as you get older, resulting in more senescent cells that don't function very well. And there seems to be some truth in that. Senescent cells accumulate with increased age in species ranging from mice to humans. Suppressing senescent cells in mice has been shown to improve their health. You may have heard of the disorder known as progeria. Children suffering from this condition undergo premature aging and die, essentially of old age, in their early teens. These children have a mutation in a gene that results in rapid cell senescence.

Shorter telomeres in humans are associated with many age-related diseases including cancer, cardiovascular disease, and dementia. But would immortality be possible if you maintain telomere length? It's not out of the question. In studies that led to a Nobel Prize in 2009, a protein called telomerase was identified that can lengthen the telomere to let cells keep on dividing. This discovery was followed by characterization of a type of worm that is, to all intents and purposes, immortal.[15] As Dr. Aziz Aboobaker of the University of Nottingham explains, "Planarian worms appear to [be able to] regenerate indefinitely by growing new muscles, skin, guts and even entire brains over and over again." So what is going on? As Aboobaker states, "Usually when stem cells divide—to heal wounds, or during reproduction or for growth—they start to show signs of aging. Our aging skin is perhaps the most visible example of this effect. Planarian worms and their stem cells are some-how able to avoid the aging process and to keep their cells dividing." The Nottingham team identified a planarian version of the gene coding for telomerase and found that at least one species of Planarian worms dramatically increase the activity of the gene that codes for telomerase when they regenerate, allowing stem cells to maintain their telomeres as they divide to replace missing tissues.

While all cells contain the gene for telomerase, it is expressed at low levels (or not at all) in most cells. It is expressed in a subset of blood cells called peripheral blood mononuclear cells (PBMC), and its activity can be measured using a relatively simple blood test; alternatively, telomere length can also be measured in various tissues. Efforts have been made to find drugs that activate telomerase, and indeed small-molecule activators of telomerase have been identified and shown in early studies to improve the apparent health status of mice. Interestingly, statins to inhibit cholesterol synthesis seem to have a telomerase-activating effect. There is evidence that growth hormones, such as human growth hormone, also activate telomerase. Meditation and adherence to the Mediterranean diet have also been associated with lengthening telomeres. A big factor is exercise, as there is growing evidence that it plays a direct role in activating telomerase—in other words, in keeping you younger.

The observation that exercise results in longer telomeres could explain the remarkable benefits of exercise in almost every area of human health. Exercise is an amazing drug; it reduces the risk of colon cancer by at least 25 percent, breast cancer by 20 percent to 40 percent, lung cancer (in smokers) by 35 percent, and skin cancer (in mice) by over 60 percent.[16] A statement from the American Heart Association in 2003 says, "Habitual physical activity prevents the development of coronary artery disease and reduces symptoms in patients with established cardiovascular disease."[17] There is also evidence that exercise reduces the risk of other chronic diseases, including type 2 diabetes, osteoporosis, obesity, and depression. It reduces blood pressure. In fact, what doesn't exercise do? It seems it keeps your telomeres long as well, which may explain some of its "magic bullet" qualities. In an article published in 2008, Tim Spector and associates at King's College London examined the effects of exercise in 2,400 sets of identical twins, and the findings were unambiguous:[18]

> People who did a moderate amount of exercise—about 100 minutes a week of an activity such as tennis, swimming or running—had telomeres that on average looked like those of someone about five or six years younger than those who did the least—about 16 minutes a week. Those who did the most—doing about three hours a week of moderate to vigorous activity—had telomeres that appeared to be about nine years younger than those who did the least. As the amount of exercise increased, the telomere length increased.

A potential downside associated with telomerase activation is that approximately 90 percent of tumor cells exhibit telomerase activity, which is consistent with their ability to divide indefinitely, so increasing cancer risk could be a concern— although it is clear that exercise does not increase cancer risk; rather, the reverse. In any event, it is likely that we will soon discover ways to prevent the accumulation of the senescent cells that makes us old. This advance could well happen within ten years. After all, the fundamental miracle is that you were born and grew to be what you are; correcting defects that appear is really just a matter of understanding the biology at the molecular level and using this understanding to reengineer tissues as they age. In the meantime, it might be a good idea to hit the gym.

Other biomarker tests that correlate with aging are also appearing. One type of epigenetic modification occurs when chemical tags known as methyl groups are attached to specific regions of genomic DNA: production of proteins from genes in those regions is inhibited. Steve Horvath of the University of California examined the relationship between DNA methylation and aging in brain, breast, skin, colon, kidney, liver, lung, and heart tissue taken from people ranging in age from newborns to 101 years old. He found 353 DNA sites where methyl groups increased or decreased with age and developed a predictive algorithm based on this data. As reported in *Genome Biology* in 2013, he found that the computed age based on DNA methylation closely predicted the age of numerous tissues to within just a few years.[19] In embryonic and induced pluripotent stem cells, the DNA methylation age proved to be near zero. Horvath says, "My goal in inventing this age-predictive tool is to help scientists improve their understanding of what speeds up and slows down the human aging process."[20] Horvath plans to examine whether DNA methylation is only a marker of aging or itself affects aging.

The onslaught on aging is gathering momentum. The observation noted in chapter 3 that the blood of young mice led to rejuvenation of the hearts of older mice has now been confirmed and extended to other organs. In three separate studies published in *Science* and *Nature* in early 2014, scientists reported that they reversed aging in the muscles and brains of old mice by running the blood of young mice—or the protein GDF11—through their veins.[21] Researchers at Harvard found that treated mice could run longer on a treadmill and had more branching blood vessels in their brains than untreated mice. GDF11 is also found in human blood. Will the observations in mice extend to people? We will certainly find out in the next ten years.

Craig Venter of genome-sequencing fame has also joined the anti-aging bandwagon, raising more than $70 million in early 2014 to start a company called Human Longevity, Inc. "Our goal is to make 100-years-old the new 60," said Peter Diamandis, CEO.[22] The company aims to scan the DNA of as many as 100,000 people a year to create a massive database that will be complemented by microbiomic, proteomic, and metabolomic data. Correlation of this data with age and presence or absence of disease is anticipated to lead to new tests and therapies that can help extend healthy human life.

Google is entering the longevity arena by forming a company called Calico.[23] Rumors have it that an objective of Calico is to extend the life of people born in the last twenty years by as much as a hundred years. Google, of course, is going to have the advantage of huge data-mining capabilities. As an early investor in 23andMe, it also has access to extensive genomic data for analysis. Other companies with similar aims are springing up with increasing frequency, backed by enormous amounts of money from private investors. As Steven Edwards, a policy analyst at the American Association for the Advancement of Science, states, "For better or worse, the practice of science in the 21st century is becoming shaped less by national priorities or by peer-review groups and more by the particular preferences of individuals with huge amounts of money."[24] And their impact seems likely to grow, given the relative decline in publicly funded research and the enormous wealth of these private individuals. A *New York Times* analysis shows that the forty or so richest science donors who have signed a pledge to give most of their fortunes to charity have assets surpassing a quarter-trillion dollars. It is not irrational to suggest that a large proportion of this money will be invested in efforts to extend the human life span, particularly the life span of the wealthy individual.

What do the next ten years hold in terms of personalized medicine and preventive care to maintain wellness? This area is set for explosive growth. Americans spend over $30 billion a year on natural health products that have no proven value,[25] and somewhat more on "functional foods" (such as probiotic yogurt) that may have benefits, but you often don't know for sure. You can imagine what consumers would spend if they knew that the food and food supplements they purchased were actually doing some good. More importantly, it would be good to know which drugs will work for you and be compatible with you. Adverse drug reactions result in approximately 10 million hospital visits per year in the U.S. and cost nearly $200 billion. Some programs just starting now will address all these issues and much, much more. One of the first is being organized by Leroy Hood of the Institute for Systems Biology in Seattle.[26] Hood is a pioneer and an extremely effective proselytizer for personalized medicine, and his study may well become a premier example of preventive medicine in the future.

If you want to know everything you can about yourself, Hood's study is for you. Participants will be extensively examined both at the molecular level and at macroscopic levels using the latest methods made possible through omic and remote-sensing technology. Their genomes will be sequenced and analyzed to identify genetic risk factors for disease and for drug compatibility. Their physical activity, heart rate, and sleep patterns will be continually monitored to ascertain health status. And every three months, microbial species in the colon, metabolites such as blood glucose (a biomarker for diabetes) and creatinine (a biomarker for kidney function), and about 100 proteins that will indicate the health of your liver, lungs, brain, and heart will be analyzed and monitored for transitions from health to disease.

Eventually, Hood plans to enroll 100,000 people, generate personal big-data clouds for all these individuals and follow them for thirty or more years. It's a measure of Hood's drive and passion, not to mention optimism, that at age seventy-five he is embarking on a study that could take thirty years to reach maturity. Transitions to common diseases such as cardiovascular diseases, cancer, and neurological diseases will occur among the test participants over this period, and by analyzing this data, Hood hopes to develop predictive models to delineate early biomarkers for disease, allowing early intervention before the disease becomes life threatening, as well as ways of detecting the resolution of disease as the participant's biomarkers return to normal. These biomarkers should also allow you to rapidly determine whether the therapy you are using to treat whatever disease you may have is, in fact, working.

All this data and subsequent analysis will lead to actionable possibilities. As Hood writes, "An actionable possibility is a feature for an individual that, if corrected, could improve wellness or avoid disease. A friend was told that he had early onset osteoporosis in his mid-30s—a disease that potentially could confine him to a wheel chair for the rest of his life. After genetic analysis, he discovered that he had a defective ability to absorb calcium. He took 20 times the normal amount of calcium for several years and returned his bone structure to normal and after about 12 years continues to remain normal on this regimen. Thus this genetic defect is actionable in that it can be corrected by taking more calcium."

Another example Hood gives concerns a physicist who began to lose interest in his work and had difficulty concentrating. As the problem continued for a considerable time, he underwent blood screening. It turned out that he was severely deficient in iron. Within days after replacement therapy, he returned to normal and resumed his former life with his typical enthusiasm. Hood believes that we have 300 to 500 of these actionable genetic variants and that many of them arise from nutritional deficiencies that can be readily corrected.

At present, the practice of medicine, particularly in hospitals, is focused on treating disease rather than preventing it. Public-health medicine and primary-care efforts by general practitioners do emphasize preventive care but mainly through encouraging exercise and healthy diets, as well as smoking cessation. This blunderbuss approach is in stark contrast to the precise, individualized information gained and used in Hood's project. The combined data generated by Hood's and other wellness initiatives will be of enormous value, as it will establish a database that can be mined to create new biomarker tests of health and disease and offer new information about the effects of environment and diet on our physical and mental states, and will also create completely new industries aimed at maintaining health and extending life. For example, data providing evidence that you're trending towards disease will lead to new therapies aimed at correcting these trends rather than treating the disease itself.

What else can we expect over the next ten years? One thing is certain: we are going to make new biological discoveries that will upset present notions about how our cells and our bodies work. The functional roles of the 98 percent of your genome that does not code for genes are an area of intense research, and it appears that a large proportion of the noncoding region of the genome plays regulatory roles for gene expression. Furthermore, approximately 90 percent of disease-associated mutations are in noncoding regions, and finding out how those mutations influence disease is likely to lead to new treatment modalities.

Other surprises are in store as we identify new biomarkers associated with disease or wellness. As discussed previously, diagnostics that use genomic, proteomic, and other data are well on their way to being of practical use. Recent studies show that the small bits of RNA called microRNA (miRNA) in body fluids such as blood can also have important diagnostic uses, such as early detection of cancer. For example, pancreatic cancer is difficult to detect until it is too late. Nicolai Schultz of the Herlev Hospital in Copenhagen has identified a panel of miRNAs in the blood that appear to be diagnostic for the presence of pancreatic cancer.[27] As Schultz states, "The test could diagnose more patients with pancreatic cancer, some of them at an early stage, and thus have a potential to increase the number of patients that can be operated on and possibly cured." Other studies suggest that miRNA screens could be used to detect ovarian cancer—another cancer that is often detected too late for effective therapy.

The potential utility of miRNA diagnostics is not limited to cancer. Eckart Meese and Andreas Keller at Saarland University have shown that by measuring the levels of twelve types of miRNA in the blood, they could predict, with 93 percent accuracy, whether or not an individual had Alzheimer's disease.[28] "At this point of our research, we are only at the beginning of a biological understanding of the miRNA pattern identified," they said in an interview. "Our results make us confident that miRNA signatures can likely play a role in the future diagnosis of Alzheimer's disease." Because Alzheimer's disease starts years before cognitive decline begins, a test for the early stages of the disease could allow early intervention, before irreparable damage is done. It is also possible that such tests could be useful to assay whether Alzheimer therapeutics are actually working by determining whether the miRNA levels revert to a normal profile.

We can expect other new types of diagnostics as well. There are stories of dogs alerting their owners to diseases such as lung cancer and breast cancer. These animals may have an ability to detect volatile organic compounds (VOCs), which can be diagnostic for cancer. Considerable work is being done to ascertain the utility of VOCs as biomarkers of disease. Peter Mazzone and his team at the Cleveland Clinic have developed a breath test for lung cancer.[29] Mazzone's test, the colorimetric sensor assay, consists of an array of pigments that change color when they come in contact with certain VOCs, and it is sensitive enough to distinguish between different types of lung cancer, including non-small cell cancer, adenocarcinoma, and squamous cell carcinoma.

New approaches to disease detection will come from unlikely sources. Pancreatic cancer, which killed Apple founder Steve Jobs, has a five-year survival rate of only 15 percent, in part because we are unable to detect early-stage disease. Fourteen-year-old Jack Andraka developed a low-cost paper strip–based test for mesothelin, a pancreatic cancer biomarker.[30] The test uses carbon nanotubes—tiny cylinders made with carbon sheets an atom thick—coated with an antibody that binds to the mesothelin. When this protein latches on to the nanotube, it changes the separation between the carbon nanotubes in a way that also changes their electrical conductivity. His invention won him the $75,000 Gordon E. Moore Award, the grand prize of the Intel International Science and Engineering Fair in 2012, when he was fifteen.

New molecular-level diagnostics for infectious disease will also appear. For example, antibiotic resistance is a major health threat, with 23,000 Americans dying from resistant strains of infections each year. A key contributor to resistance is the over-use of antibiotics, particularly to treat viral infections, which antibiotics cannot affect. Because it can be hard to tell the difference between a viral and a bacterial infection, physicians often write prescriptions for antibiotics, just in case. In many countries, patients buy them over the counter, just to make sure. At Duke University, Geoffrey Ginsburg and his team have detected different gene-expression profiles in response to viral infections as opposed to bacterial infections.[31] Ginsburg's test boasts a 90 percent accuracy rate in identifying a viral respiratory infection and can return results within twelve hours, compared with the days that traditional test results take.

Other new advances, especially for treating cancer, are likely as we achieve greater understanding and control of the immune system. As detailed in chapter 5, great advances are being made by manipulating the immune system to treat blood cancers such as leukemias, and it is likely that in the next decade, similar methods will be developed to treat solid cancers such as lung and breast cancer. Creating these treatments will require the development of ways to defeat the ability of these cancer cells to suppress the immune system, but efforts are under way to do just that. At Stanford University, Irving Weissman and his team have developed an antibody that prompts the immune system to recognize and attack cancer cells.[32] The ability of cancer cells to avoid recognition by the immune system comes partly from a protein called CD47, which sends a "don't eat me" signal to macrophages—the white blood cells that destroy pathogenic invaders. By blocking CD47, Weissman's antibody allows the macrophages to attack the cancer cells and in turn mobilize the body's entire immune response against the cancer. What's exciting about Weissman's work is that CD47 isn't specific to any particular cancer: "What we've shown is that CD47 isn't just important on leukemias and lymphomas," says Weissman. "It's on every single human primary tumor that we tested."

Surprises are definitely going to come as we understand more about the brain and how it functions. In 2013, Michael McConnell at the Salk Institute for Biological Studies discovered that our neurons vary to a striking degree: as many as 40 percent of neurons exhibit large chunks of deleted or duplicated DNA (known as copy number variants, or CNVs) as compared to a "standard" neuron.[33] As McConnell told *ScienceDaily*, "The thing about neurons is that, unlike skin cells, they don't turn over, and they interact with each other. They form these big complex circuits, where one cell that has CNVs that make it different can potentially have network-wide influence in a brain." Spontaneous CNVs have been linked with schizophrenia and autism, so developing an understanding of how CNVs form could clarify origins of mental health disorders.

As you may already have come to appreciate, technology never ends, and we are going to get additional surprises as new technologies come online. Three-dimensional (3D) printing, now in its infancy, is going to have a profound impact. Its applications couldn't be more personalized. In March 2013, a man in the northeastern U.S. had 75 percent of his skull replaced by a 3D-printed polymer implant, designed with the help of CT scans.[34] Using an inkjet-type device, Keith Martin and his team at the University of Cambridge have successfully layered living retinal cells.[35] Said Martin, "This is the first time that cells from the adult central nervous system have been successfully printed. We've demonstrated that you can take cells from the retina and you can effectively separate them out. We can print those cells out in any pattern we like, and we've shown that those cells can survive and thrive." Although this research is still in its early stages, it points to the potential for sculpted tissues customized to the patient. Martin suggests that these techniques will lead to eventual cures for macular degeneration and glaucoma, the two leading causes of blindness in developed countries. It is not hard to imagine the combination of 3D printing techniques and stem cell technology leading to an ability to grow organs outside your body, for subsequent implantation.

Advances in stem cell technology will also lead to new drugs. For example, Gabsang Lee of the Johns Hopkins Institute for Cell Engineering extracted skin cells from an individual suffering from Riley-Day syndrome, a rare genetic disorder affecting sensory nerves.[36] People with Riley-Day have frequent vomiting crises, problems with speech and movement, difficulty swallowing, inappropriate perception of heat, pain, and taste, unstable blood pressure, and gastrointestinal problems. Using the induced pluripotent stem cell approach, Lee and his team coaxed those skin cells into becoming neurons. They were then able to screen thousands of drugs to see which ones would make the neurons express higher levels of the genes that were not produced in adequate amounts. "Because we could study the nerve cells directly, we could for the first time see exactly what was going wrong in this disease," said Lee. They ultimately identified a compound that shows promise for stopping or reversing Riley-Day syndrome.

Personalized approaches to health care are also going to be extended to more tailored treatment of the very young and the very old. As noted by the Institute of Medicine, "The majority of drugs prescribed for children—50 to 75 percent— have not been tested in pediatric populations."[37] In essence, we treat children as if they are little adults, usually changing dose levels according to their weight. Adults and children have "profound anatomical, physiological, and developmental differences," which translate into differences in how they metabolize drugs—meaning that results from drug trials on adults may not apply to children at all.

Variability is a huge problem for the elderly. John Sloan, a physician who cares for geriatric patients, writes that "the fragile elderly are different from one another in all sorts of ways."[38] He cited kidney function as an example:

> As you get older, particularly when you get really old, two things happen. One, kidney function gets worse. So an average eighty-year-old patient will definitely have worse kidney function than she did when she was twenty. But thing number two is that the older you get, the wider the range of kidney function gets. Kidney function becomes heterogeneous. Result: blood levels of kidney-filtered drugs are heterogeneous. One elderly person has kidney function close to that of a normal forty-year-old; another one has awful, barely functioning kidneys. Give a kidney-filtered drug at its textbook dose to the first one, everything is cool. Give it to the second one, the blood level is through the roof and side effects have her flat on her back.

For the fragile elderly, this variability can extend to many organs, making prescribing the right dosage of a drug a huge challenge. As a result, many patients are overmedicated, and serious adverse drug reactions can be dismissed as just another consequence of aging. Compounding the problem is that these patients are usually on several drugs at once, and they can interact with each other to produce new problems. Accurate biomarkers to monitor the therapeutic effects of drugs in this population are desperately needed to achieve the right doses of the right drugs and avoid adverse drug interactions.

At the beginning of this chapter, the democratization of medicine was mentioned as a probable event resulting from molecularly based medicine over the next ten years. But what does this mean? It means that through the availability of inexpensive, accurate, molecular-level diagnostic tests, consumers will be able to get much more definitive information regarding their own health, which will allow them to become much more actively involved in managing it. Patients will no longer be passive recipients of diagnosis and treatment by the medical profession. Health care is moving from hospitals and clinics to the home, into the hands of you, the consumer, as personalized medicine technologies improve self-monitoring and your understanding of your body in health and disease. There are risks and many regulatory issues, but one thing is certain: the democratization and demystification of health care is starting to happen.

There is one large—and unanswered—question in all these conjectures about what may happen over the coming decade: Will all this information make any difference on a population-wide level? Will individuals change their behavior when they can get accurate, predictive information about their health status? This is not an idle question: current evidence suggests that many of us won't. We all know we should follow a balanced diet low in saturated fats and get more exercise, and smokers have all been told the health risks of cigarettes, but most of us indulge in behaviors that we know are harmful to our health. As health-care editor Paul Cerrato wrote in a commentary for *InformationWeek*,[39] "Most people want to see a doctor only when something breaks down, and then they expect a pill or procedure to make things right, just as they expect their car mechanic to fix their cars. Health care for most Americans is about having someone else 'make it better,' not about personal responsibility." Google's attempt to launch a personal health-record product, Google Health, was shut down after a few years of low uptake, with the company announcing on its blog, "There has been adoption among certain groups of users like tech-savvy patients and their caregivers, and more recently fitness and wellness enthusiasts. But we haven't found a way to translate that limited usage into widespread adoption in the daily health routines of millions of people."[40] It is entirely possible that a similar situation will evolve for personalized medicine, in which an elite few who actually use the information available gain considerable benefits but the majority do not. It will be interesting to see how this scenario evolves.

So within the next ten years, personalized medicine will be available to you and will be front and center in the medical scene. It will surely create unrealistic expectations and will be the subject of many portentous editorials saying that the hype far exceeds reality. It will place enormous strains on the medical system as patients become increasingly empowered by real information that they will want acted upon immediately and as doctors try to adjust to a new environment where many of their present skills become outmoded. It may well cause a large number of healthy people to become sick as they try to correct trivial problems they detect. It will cause enormous growth in the health-maintenance industry, which will become the biggest industry of all time. And it will increasingly cater to the desire to change ourselves in ways that make us smarter or better looking or younger. Human evolution won't be practiced in the Darwinian sense anymore: we'll do it to ourselves.

7

THE GENIE
IS OUT OF
THE BOTTLE

SO, WHERE ARE WE? In the previous six chapters, you have seen how the development and application of modern science over the last 400 years have led to an understanding of everything from planetary motion to the innermost workings of the cells in your body. You have learned about many of the bits and pieces that you're made of, what they do, and how you can measure them, resulting in the "molecular you." We have seen how the advent of the digital age allows us to store all this information electronically, and how analysis of the "digital you" embodied by this massive data cloud can identify biomarkers that provide an incredibly accurate picture of your state of health and disease. Remote-sensing devices can now analyze every breath you take and every beat of your heart and alert you well before you pass your best before, or rest in peace, date. Through social media, you will soon be able to share these intimate details with sympathetic listeners suffering from disorders just like yours, compare your digital selves to find the most effective therapies that should work for you, and locate where these are available. Taken together, these advances are driving massive changes in the practice of medicine as we know it today.

But that's only the beginning of the potential disruptions molecular medicine may cause.

Let's explore the near future first. Chapter 6 described what might happen during the next ten years, and it seems pretty exciting. Ten years from now, cancer will be managed much better than it is today. Detection of causative "driver" genes in your cancer genome should allow for a personalized cocktail of drugs to be administered to you to cure or control the particular cancer you have. Blood tests to detect pre-cancerous conditions and very early manifestations of cancer should be routine, allowing for effective treatment before cancers metastasize to other parts of the body. Increasingly sophisticated imaging techniques will detect the extent of your cancers more readily, leading to more complete removal of cancer cells during surgery. Today's anticancer drugs will be augmented by "smart" nanomedicines that are specifically designed to kill cancer cells and avoid healthy tissue. Perhaps most importantly, we will have ways to turn your immune system on so that it recognizes and destroys many forms of cancer. In short, a remarkably powerful array of weapons are coming online to contain and cure cancer.

How about cardiovascular disease, the other major killer in Western society, leading to heart attacks and strokes and accounting for nearly 50 percent of all deaths? Again, in the near future, we should see major advances to the point that most manifestations of heart disease will be treatable. Heart failure, the end-stage of heart disease, could be treatable, although that treatment will rely on advances in methods for rejuvenating aged hearts trending towards failure, such as ways to make heart stem cells "younger." These advances might include the human analogue of the GDF11 protein. We should have much more sophisticated techniques to predict and prevent strokes: simple blood tests to give warning signals of such events so that appropriate action can be taken. However, treatment of brain damage after it has occurred as a result of a stroke may not be that much better unless we can develop new ways to remove dead brain tissue and stimulate new neuron growth to replace dead cells.

Focused attacks based on molecular-level understanding of genetic diseases such as cystic fibrosis, Huntington's disease, or Alzheimer's disease should soon result in improved treatments. As molecular-level understanding increases, rapid advances become possible; when you know what is causing the problem, the path to a solution is much clearer.

The rapid advances in accurate diagnostics that can be anticipated in the near future, and their availability to you, will challenge the medical establishment's role as the gatekeeper of medical advances, because knowledge and power will be passed to you, the consumer. For example, the current fifteen-year wait time for a new medical advance to reach the doctor's office—to reach you—will not be tenable when you know with certainty what disorder you have, and have done your research as to which therapy is most appropriate to you and where it is available.

Let's look at a future scenario: You wake up one day feeling ill. You're very tired and somewhat nauseous. On most days when you feel like this, you open up your smartphone and find a pop-up suggesting that you drink a bit less alcohol and get more sleep. But today your smartphone suggests you run a blood analysis, because the onboard sensors on your smartwatch or bracelet have detected that things aren't right: perhaps your temperature has risen or your heart is beating a little faster. You pull out a disposable needle and prick your finger, just like diabetics do routinely, and daub a drop of blood on a disposable sensor that you plug into your smartphone. Instantly, a thousand proteins and metabolites in your blood are measured and compared against your normal levels. Meanwhile, your smartwatch and other onboard sensors are relaying your blood pressure, temperature, heart rate, body weight, respiration, and other data to be uploaded to the latest version of your digital data cloud—your digital you. Through your voice-activated personal data assistant (a.k.a. a super smartphone—Siri will work better by then), you ask your digital self, "What's wrong with me, and what should I do?" Armed with the data, your digital self answers, "We are coming down with a type of flu that has a 98 percent probability of being the same as a local strain that has been recently detected in other people in our vicinity." It works out the most appropriate individualized therapy for you, finding drugs that will work for you and that won't induce some nasty side effect. It then notifies the nearest pharmacy to prepare your individualized therapy. You pick it up, and by the next day, you're feeling your usual self again.

A second scenario: You are walking at what is usually a comfortable pace but suddenly become breathless. You sit down but can't seem to catch your breath. In this case, your onboard monitoring systems are picking up warning signs—abnormal heart rhythm, low blood oxygen, and other signs pointing to heart failure. The information is relayed to emergency services, and your smartphone informs you that an ambulance is on its way, arriving soon enough so that emergency care, such as oxygen, can be given. On arrival at the emergency room, you find that the appropriate drugs for your condition have already been prepared for you, using input from your digital you to decide which drugs will work for you, which dosage to use, and which drugs to avoid. If conditions such as atrial fibrillation have set in, blood-clot–dissolving agents will be administered before more serious problems, such as stroke, can occur.

A third scenario: Perhaps you develop type 1 diabetes. Cells are taken from your skin or some other source, and the differentiation process that caused those cells to become skin cells is reversed, yielding stem cells capable of becoming any cell in your body. They are then induced to become beta cells capable of producing insulin in response to high blood-glucose levels. These beta cells are grown in tissue culture to the required amounts and then injected intravenously into your body, where they seed in your liver and other locations, sense the glucose levels in your circulation, release insulin as needed, and resolve your diabetes. Or you find that you're trending to type 2 diabetes; you feel fine, but your onboard sensors have noted warning signs that your blood-sugar levels are rising. You receive increasingly insistent messages—a pop-up every time you open your computer or use your smartphone—that you must alter your lifestyle. You will be told to get off the subway one stop earlier or not to go back to the buffet table. You will eventually succumb to these intrusions as increasingly dire warnings flash up indicating the number of years of your life that are in jeopardy and the limbs you may lose as the diabetes progresses.

Personalized medicine heralds the start of an age of maintaining health, as opposed to treating sickness, and personalized medicine will become the major industry of the future, particularly as the health-maintenance industry increasingly engages in an anti-aging agenda. We see many signs of this now. Thirty years ago, fitness centers were almost unknown; today, if a hotel doesn't have good workout facilities, guests are irate. The health and anti-aging centers of the near future will be something to behold. There will be detailed genomic, proteomic, metabolomic, microbiomic, and vital-sign analyses to begin with, followed by daily exercise routines and diets devised specifically for you. Motivation will be provided by very precise molecular measurements that will show definitively when you make even minor progress. From standing desks at work to regular visits to a health center, very few of us will spend less than an hour a day maintaining our health. Prehab instead of rehab will be normal rather than unusual. Who would look askance at somebody in rehab for two hours a day to recover from the effects of a stroke? Far better to spend an hour a day in prehab and avoid the stroke in the first place.

What else does the near future hold? Certainly, personalized medicine will be creating havoc within the medical profession. The role of doctors in making diagnoses will be increasingly supplanted by computer analyses of the digital you. Accurate diagnoses combined with advanced imaging techniques and analyses of genomic and other data in the digital you will mean that safe and effective treatments will be readily identified. Thus the role of doctors will be in transition, as it has been for some time. Fifty years ago, doctors cared for people who were really unwell: 80 percent of their job was looking after the dying or seriously ill. Today, the treatment of chronic disease has become the norm. Care of type-2 diabetes, high blood pressure, arthritis, and cancer survivors takes up the majority of time. As these chronic disorders become increasingly controlled through a molecularly based, personalized approach, and as diagnosis and treatment are largely decided by analysis of the digital you, only complex and severe problems will need the doctor. So what will doctors be doing?

Two scenarios are possible. Those who do not have access to a doctor—or advanced health care—will find the playing field dramatically leveled. Relatively inexpensive omic data—potentially in the range of $100 for a complete analysis—and free online analyses available through the Internet will enable patients around the world to access state-of-the-art diagnostic resources. This information, combined with Internet searches and social media such as PatientsLikeMe, CureTogether, and other disease-specific websites, will also make it possible for you to discover what the most appropriate treatment is and where it is available. You'll be able to do some cost-comparison shopping as well as check references from satisfied (or unsatisfied) customers. Having decided on the best, most cost-effective therapy, you will then make an appointment and travel arrangements to get treated.

An alternative scenario—and one that people with adequate health plans and access to doctors will tend to move to: You will still have a doctor, but you will rely on him or her to prevent you getting ill, rather than to treat you after you become unwell. Your doctor will likely be associated with a health-maintenance center that you belong to, and it is likely you will pay your doctor according to his or her success in keeping you well. Your doctor will help keep you well by assisting you not only with the latest ways of gathering important personal data but also by helping you analyze and interpret your digital self and by advising you on the most appropriate course of action. You will probably fire your doctor if you get sick too often. This is a novel concept—paying doctors only for effective treatments and recommendations. Takes one back to the halcyon days of ancient Mesopotamia: according to Hammurabi's code of laws, physicians who performed surgery were held responsible for errors or failures. If a freeman died as a result of surgery, the physician could have his fingers cut off. If a slave died as a result of surgery, the physician had to replace the slave with one of equal value. In any event, we may not need so many doctors with the training they presently have. The expert systems that interpret our personal data cloud will bear a lot of the load. But doctors who play the role of health coach will be very much in demand to manage and optimize our health in the same way that we now use financial professionals to manage and grow our investments or lawyers to manage and solve our legal problems.

But let's move on to the really interesting bit: what's in the cards for personalized medicine over the longer term—say, fifty years from now? Here we realize that the genie is certainly out of the bottle: a molecular-level understanding of ourselves has many consequences, and not all of them are unambiguously wonderful.

Right now, the efforts humankind has made to understand and cure our various ailments are starting to show signs of working. As Winston Churchill said after Britain won its first battle in the Second World War: "This is not the end, this is not even the beginning of the end, but it is, perhaps, the end of the beginning."

So what is the end? This question is difficult to answer because the sky is the limit. We are only now coming to appreciate the incredible power that the focused application of science and technology can have on our individual selves. Only slightly more than 400 years after the initial attacks on magical thinking by Galileo and Newton, we are starting to come to grips with what we're made of, how it's put together, and how it can be fixed. Progress is accelerating wildly. Approximately 90 percent of scientists who ever lived are alive today. A large proportion of them are working to bring better health to all. Until 1900, human knowledge doubled approximately every century. By the end of the Second World War, knowledge was doubling every twenty-five years. Today, nanotechnology knowledge is doubling every two years, clinical knowledge every eighteen months, and total human knowledge every thirteen months. IBM is projecting the doubling of knowledge as the Internet is built out to be as short as every twelve hours. Knowledge drives technology drives change, and we are hurtling blindly into future change at an ever-increasing rate.

So if you think the rate of change now is way too fast, fasten your seatbelts. The rate of change is going to get a lot faster, particularly in medicine. The changes enabled by new knowledge will be aided and abetted by the fact that when it comes right down to it, we all want to escape from the natural order of things. The signs are all around us. If your hip or knee wears out, replace it. If your heart slows down, put in a pacemaker. If you can't hear, get a hearing aid. If you can't get an erection, use Viagra. Now it's about to get much better—or worse, depending on your point of view. It is starting, obviously enough, with diagnosis and treatment of disease, and there is no way you can argue that this is anything other than good. Clearly, your cancer should be identified and treated in a way that actually affects the cancer and does not harm the rest of you. Clearly, it is ridiculous that after an operation to remove a cancer, you have to wait for three months or six months to see whether the disease is returning: you should have a simple blood test to map your progress on a weekly or daily basis. Clearly, you should not wait until a disease is advanced before you treat it; you should know well ahead that you are trending towards disease and take appropriate action. Clearly, you shouldn't take a drug that doesn't work to treat your disease; you should use only drugs that work on you and don't harm you. It is all so clear, but there are many concerns.

Chief among these concerns is the probability that the rate of increase of knowledge and the associated rate of improvement in technology is a double-edged sword. On one hand, as applied to your health, the potential benefits are legion. On the other hand, as Donald Rumsfeld would put it, there are many unknown unknowns that could surprise us. Stanislaw Ulam, in a tribute to the great mathematician and physicist John von Neumann more than fifty years ago,[1] recollected a conversation "centered on the ever accelerating progress of technology and changes in the mode of human life which gives the appearance of approaching some essential singularity in the history of the race beyond which human affairs, as we know them, could not continue." Many serious thinkers today have similar concerns. Raymond Kurzweil, who is a director of engineering at Google, who received the National Medal of Technology and Innovation in 1999 (America's highest honor in technology), and whom PBS named as one of the sixteen revolutionaries who made America,[2] published a book in 2005 entitled *The Singularity Is Near: When Humans Transcend Biology*, predicting a "technological singularity" before 2050.[3] This singularity is defined as a point where progress is so rapid it outstrips humans' ability to comprehend it. Once that singularity has been reached, Kurzweil predicts machine intelligence that is much more powerful than human intelligence. What this would mean for the world, and our place in it, is not at all clear.

The global consequences of rapid technological change such as those suggested by Kurzweil are arguable, and some would dismiss them as science fiction. However, what is not arguable is that as a result of dramatically improving technologies, much more definitive information is becoming available about how we are made, what is wrong with each of us, and what will work for each of us, and that information in turn is opening the door to using new understanding of biology to cure our diseases, correct our defects, and extend our lives. It can be expected that these efforts will become increasingly intensive and that the rush towards personalized medicine in the near future will be an expression of this. There is an enormous demand for these services because we feel that we are captives of so many things we cannot fix or control. We are captives of disease, pain, and disability—particularly as we get older. We are captives of our bodies—robust or not, attractive or ugly. We are captives of life itself; as Jim Morrison, lead singer for the Doors, put it: "No one gets out of here alive."

Thus the endgame of personalized medicine will be an ability to not only fix diseases we may have but also extend our lives and "improve" ourselves. The list of improvements we may want is endless: to make ourselves more intelligent, more attractive, more athletic, younger—the wish list can be pretty extensive. Whether this power will come in 50 years or 100 years can be debated, but what cannot be ignored is that in less than 500 years, a blink of an eye in evolutionary time, we have come to the rapidly expanding understanding of life that we have today. It would be delusionary to deny the potential for extending our life spans and fixing our imperfections. As our wishes come true, fundamental drivers in our civilization will be perturbed. The fact that we are going to die in the not too distant future drives a lot of our behavior; it drives a search to understand why we're here, why we do what we do, and where we're going, particularly after we die. This search has not been particularly fruitful, so we invent constructs such as nationality and culture and religion and invest these with a significance and importance that is not entirely rational yet makes sense of our lives and provides a set of rules to live by.

The probable reality is that we are exquisitely evolved survival machines, whose objective is survival of the species, and nothing more. Every attribute we have can be fitted into that framework. And in the Darwinian scheme of things, once we have procreated and raised our young, evolution has no further use for us, and that's when we age and die. But our search for meaning in life will change significantly if we are able to eliminate pain and suffering and extend life indefinitely: we still won't understand what the hell is going on, but it won't be as pressing an issue if pain and death are not around the next corner. Eat, drink, and be merry, for tomorrow you may not die.

Personalized medicine that leads to dramatically extended life spans is an amazing, and sobering, prospect, and it is here that the darker side of the genie we have let out of the bottle begins to emerge. From the individual point of view, of course, this promise is wonderful. We may no longer be subject to the impersonal cruelty of Darwinian pressures, no longer have to die within some predetermined timeframe, and no longer have to endure the pain of terminal disease. The prospect of genetic surgery suggests the advent of designer bodies: If we are able to replace old stem cells with new ones that are younger, why not change the genetic code so that your eyes will gradually change to that piercing blue that you've always wanted? Why not code for that larger penis, or those longer legs, or neurons that work a little better? But we had better be careful, because we are changing the natural order of things and there will be repercussions.

From an environmental point of view, of course, the ability to extend life significantly, say to 150 years or more, would be an unmitigated disaster. Technology has already dramatically extended our life spans over the last 200 years, from 40 years in 1800 to 80 years in 2012. The fact that there are so many of us is at the heart of all environmental problems, and increased life spans certainly won't help. Even more of a problem will be the lack of renewal and the frustration of younger generations when parents and grandparents don't die off. And what of super-rich captains of industry or dictators who just won't go away? Another 100 years of Donald Trump or Robert Mugabe? Or prolongation of ancient credos that keep women subjugated and old wounds festering, never healed by the renewal process inherent in death? There is little doubt that revolution will be in the air.

So the future will be interesting. For the readers of this book, if you want to enhance your health, the way is clear. First, exercise, eat healthful food, and don't smoke. You should pay attention to this advice: it applies to all of us. Second, the molecular-level information you need to find out your own risks, diagnose your particular ailments, and discover the best treatments just for you is coming online. You should pay attention to this opportunity: it may save your life. Third, we are merrily changing the natural order of things to ensure survival of the individual as opposed to the species, with not a clue as to the consequences. You should pay attention to this phenomenon: it could lead to the end of the human race as we know it. You can't stop our mad dash into the future, but you really do need to know what is happening. Personalized molecularly based medicine is driving the major revolution of your time.

We are all pioneers in a brave new world.

ACKNOWLEDGMENTS

I HAVE MANY people to thank who helped me to write this book.

First and foremost is Nancy Flight, love of my life, who after hearing me talk on the benefits of personalized medicine recognized a potential book and found a way to get me to write it. Without her this book would not have happened. I thank her for that, for her incisive advice and encouragement and so much more. Next, I thank my collaborators on the Personalized Medicine Initiative: Mike Burgess, Martin Dawes, Rob Fraser, David Huntsman, Bruce McManus, and Jim Russell. It has been a remarkable privilege and education working with such consummate professionals and, even better, an enormous amount of fun as we scheme to change the medical system. I also thank my children, Jane Cullis and Jeffrey Cullis, for their pointed, intelligent, and gratefully received criticisms. Lastly, I thank my editors: Iva Cheung, who helped enormously in the initial stages of putting this manuscript together, and Catherine Plear, who was of tremendous help in transforming my fevered jottings into a manuscript that is much more readable.

With all this help, I should have produced a much better book. Any errors, omissions, or terminological inexactitudes are, of course, purely my fault. I do hope, however, that the central theme of this book—that personalized medicine is and will be the major revolution of our time—is clear. We do live in exciting times.

SOURCES

CHAPTER 1

1. Kanu Chatterjee et al., "Doxorubicin Cardiomyopathy," *Cardiology* 115, no. 2 (January 2010): 155–62.

2. Chuenjid Kongkaew, Peter R. Noyce, and Darren M. Ashcroft, "Hospital Admissions Associated with Adverse Drug Reactions: A Systematic Review of Prospective Observational Studies," *The Annals of Pharmacotherapy* 42 (2008): 1017–25.

3. Robin McKie, "Growing Lifespan Shows No Sign of Slowing, but Don't Expect Immortality," *The Observer*, March 6, 2011, http://www.theguardian .com/society/2011/mar/06/lifespan-mortality-health-diabetes.

4. Qiuping Gu, Charles F. Dillon, and Vicki L. Burt, "Prescription Drug Use Continues to Increase: U.S. Prescription Drug Data for 2007– 2008," *NCHS Data Briefs*, no. 42 (2010), http://www.cdc.gov/nchs/data/ databriefs/db42.htm.

5. Jason Lazarou, Bruce H. Pomeranz, and Paul N. Corey, "Incidence of Adverse Drug Reactions in Hospitalized Patients," *Journal of the American Medical Association* 279, no. 15 (April 15, 1998): 1200.

6. Lorna Hazell and Saad A.W. Shakir, "Under-Reporting of Adverse Drug Reactions: A Systematic Review," *Drug Safety: An International Journal of Medical Toxicology and Drug Experience* 29, no. 5 (January 2006): 385–96.

7. Brian B. Spear, Margo Heath-Chiozzi, and Jeffrey Huff, "Clinical Application of Pharmacogenetics," *Trends in Molecular Medicine* 7, no. 5 (May 5, 2001): 201–4.

8. Cleveland Clinic, "Health and Prevention: Statin Medications and Heart Disease," *Cleveland Clinic,* http://my.clevelandclinic.org/ heart/ prevention/risk-factors/cholesterol/statin-medications-heart -disease.aspx.

9. Huabing Zhang et al., "Discontinuation of Statins in Routine Care Settings: A Cohort Study," *Annals of Internal Medicine* 158, no. 7 (April 2, 2013): 526–34.

10. Lara M. Mangravite et al., "A Statin-Dependent QTL for GATM Expression Is Associated with Statin-Induced Myopathy," *Nature* 502, no. 7471 (October 17, 2013): 377–80.

11. Siddhartha Mukherjee, *The Emperor of All Maladies: A Biography of Cancer* (New York, NY: Scribner, 2011), pp. 35–37.

12. Y. Li, R.B. Womer, and J.H. Silber, "Predicting Cisplatin Ototoxicity in Children: The Influence of Age and the Cumulative Dose," *European Journal of Cancer* 40, no. 16 (November 2004): 2445–51.

13. Matthew Herper, "The Truly Staggering Cost of Inventing New Drugs," *Forbes*, February 10, 2012, http://www.forbes.com/sites/matthewherper/2012/02/10/the-truly-staggering-cost-of-inventing-new-drugs/.

CHAPTER 2

1. Stephen Bent, "Herbal Medicine in the United States: Review of Efficacy, Safety, and Regulation: Grand Rounds at University of California, San Francisco Medical Center," *Journal of General Internal Medicine* 23, no. 6 (June 2008): 854–59.

2. "Charles Darwin's Health," *Wikipedia,* accessed September 12, 2014, http://en.wikipedia.org/wiki/Charles_Darwin's_health.

3. J.B. Durand, A.B. Abchee, and R. Roberts, "Molecular and Clinical Aspects of Inherited Cardiomyopathies," *Annals of Medicine* 27, no. 3 (June 1995): 311–17, http://www.ncbi.nlm.nih.gov/pubmed/7546620; Shiro Kamakura, "Epidemiology of Brugada Syndrome in Japan and Rest of the World," *Journal of Arrhythmia* 29, no. 2 (April 1, 2013): 52–55; B.J. Maron et al., "Prevalence of Hypertrophic Cardiomyopathy in a General Population of Young Adults: Echocardiographic Analysis of 4111 Subjects in the CARDIA Study," *Circulation* 92, no. 4 (August 15, 1995): 785–89; Carlo Napolitano, Silvia G. Priori, and Raffaella Bloise, "Catecholaminergic Polymorphic Ventricular Tachycardia," in *GeneReviews,* ed. Roberta A. Pagon (Seattle, WA: University of Washington, 2014); Peter J. Schwartz et al., "Prevalence of the Congenital Long-QT Syndrome," *Circulation* 120, no. 18 (November 3, 2009): 1761–67.

4. Robert F. Service, "A $1000 Genome by 2013?," *Science News*, July 2011, http://news.sciencemag.org/math/2011/07/1000-genome-2013.

CHAPTER 3

1. Alok Jha, "Breakthrough Study Overturns Theory of 'Junk DNA' in Genome," *The Guardian*, September 5, 2012, http://www.theguardian.com/science/2012/sep/05/genes-genome-junk-dna-encode.

2. Jonah Riddell et al., "Reprogramming Committed Murine Blood Cells to Induced Hematopoietic Stem Cells with Defined Factors," *Cell* 157, no. 3 (April 24, 2014): 549–64.

3. J.B. Gurdon and V. Uehlinger, "'Fertile' Intestine Nuclei," *Nature* 210, no. 5042 (June 18, 1966): 1240–41, http://www.ncbi.nlm.nih.gov/pubmed/5967799.

4. K.H. Campbell et al., "Sheep Cloned by Nuclear Transfer from a Cultured Cell Line," *Nature* 380, no. 6569 (March 7, 1996): 64–66.

5. Francesco S. Loffredo et al., "Growth Differentiation Factor 11 Is a Circulating Factor That Reverses Age-Related Cardiac Hypertrophy," *Cell* 153, no. 4 (May 9, 2013): 828–39.

6. Michael Specter, "Germs Are Us," *The New Yorker*, October 22, 2012, http://www.newyorker.com/magazine/2012/10/22/germs-are-us.

7. Ilseung Cho and Martin J. Blaser, "The Human Microbiome: At the Interface of Health and Disease," *Nature Reviews: Genetics* 13, no. 4 (April 2012): 260–70.

8. N. Lender et al., "Review Article: Associations between Helicobacter Pylori and Obesity—an Ecological Study," *Alimentary Pharmacology and Therapeutics* 40, no. 1 (July 2014): 24–31.

9. Ilseung Cho et al., "Antibiotics in Early Life Alter the Murine Colonic Microbiome and Adiposity," *Nature* 488, no. 7413 (August 30, 2012): 621–26.

10. E.J. Videlock and F. Cremonini, "Meta-Analysis: Probiotics in Antibiotic-Associated Diarrhoea," *Alimentary Pharmacology and Therapeutics* 35, no. 12 (June 2012): 1355–69.

11. "*Clostridium Difficile* Infection," *Centers for Disease Control and Prevention*, accessed July 26, 2014, http://www.cdc.gov/hai/organisms/cdiff/cdiff_infect.html.

12. J.L. Anderson, R.J. Edney, and K. Whelan, "Systematic Review: Faecal Microbiota Transplantation in the Management of Inflammatory Bowel Disease," *Alimentary Pharmacology and Therapeutics* 36, no. 6 (September 2012): 503–16.

13. David E. Elliott and Joel V. Weinstock, "Helminthic Therapy: Using Worms to Treat Immune-Mediated Disease," *Advances in Experimental Medicine and Biology* 666 (January 2009): 157–66, http://www.ncbi.nlm.nih.gov/pubmed/20054982.

CHAPTER 4

1. Bala Murali Venkatesan and Rashid Bashir, "Nanopore Sensors for Nucleic Acid Analysis," *Nature Nanotechnology* 6, no. 10 (October 2011): 615–24.

2. Scott D. McCulloch and Thomas A. Kunkel, "The Fidelity of DNA Synthesis by Eukaryotic Replicative and Translesion Synthesis Polymerases," *Cell Research* 18, no. 1 (January 2008): 148–61.

3. J.N. Adkins et al., "Toward a Human Blood Serum Proteome: Analysis by Multidimensional Separation Coupled with Mass Spectrometry," *Molecular and Cellular Proteomics* 1, no. 12 (November 15, 2002): 947–55.

4. Andrew J. Percy et al., "Standardized Protocols for Quality Control of MRM-Based Plasma Proteomic Workflows," *Journal of Proteome Research* 12, no. 1 (January 4, 2013): 222–33.

5. "Why Are Larger Sized Hard Drives Consistently Getting Cheaper?," *Record Nations*, accessed July 29, 2014, http://www.recordnations.com/articles/bigger-hard-drives/.

6. Mike Orcutt, "Bases to Bytes," *MIT Technology Review*, 2012, http://www.technologyreview.com/graphiti/427720/bascs-to-bytes/.

7. *PatientsLikeMe,* http://www.patientslikeme.com/.

8. *CureTogether,* http://www.curetogether.com.

9. *PXE International,* http://www.pxe.org/.

10. Sarah C.P. Williams, "Mining Consumers' Web Searches Can Reveal Unreported Side Effects of Drugs, Researchers Say," *Stanford Bio-X*, 2013, https://biox.stanford.edu/highlight/mining-consumers'-web-searches-can-reveal-unreported-side-effects-drugs -researchers-say.

11. W. Yang et al., "Economic Costs of Diabetes in the U.S. in 2012," *Diabetes Care* 36, no. 4 (April 2013): 1033–46.

12. "Heart Disease Facts," *Centers for Disease Control and Prevention*, 2014, http://www.cdc.gov/heartdisease/facts.htm.

CHAPTER 5

1. Jon Cohen, "Examining His Own Body, Stanford Geneticist Stops Diabetes in Its Tracks," *Science News*, March 2012, http://news.sciencemag.org/biology/2012/03/examining-his-own-body-stanford-geneticist-stops-diabetes-its-tracks.

2. Hangwi Tang and Jennifer Hwee Kwoon Ng, "Googling for a Diagnosis—Use of Google as a Diagnostic Aid: Internet Based Study," *BMJ (Clinical Research Ed.)* 333, no. 7579 (December 2, 2006): 1143–45.

3. Eta S. Berner and Mark L. Graber, "Overconfidence as a Cause of Diagnostic Error in Medicine," *The American Journal of Medicine* 121, no. 5 Suppl (May 2008): S2–23.

4. Maria Fuller, Peter J. Meikle, and John J. Hopwood, "Epidemiology of Lysosomal Storage Diseases: An Overview," in *Fabry Disease: Perspectives from 5 Years of FOS*, ed. Atul Mehta, Michael Beck, and Gere Sunder-Plassmann (Oxford: Oxford PharmaGenesis, 2006), http://www.ncbi.nlm.nih.gov/books/NBK11603/.

5. "Table of Pharmacogenomic Biomarkers in Drug Labeling," *Food and Drug Administration*, http://www.fda.gov/drugs/scienceresearch/researchareas/pharmacogenetics/ucm083378.htm.

6. "Gene Responsible for Acetaminophen-Induced Liver Injury Identified," *ScienceDaily*, May 11, 2009, http://www.sciencedaily.com/releases/2009/05/090504171943.htm.

7. Svati H. Shah and Deepak Voora, "Warfarin Dosing and VKORC1/CYP2C9," *Medscape*, accessed July 28, 2014, http://emedicine.medscape.com/article/1733331-overview.

8. Tom Lynch and Amy Price, "The Effect of Cytochrome P450 Metabolism on Drug Response, Interactions, and Adverse Effects," *American Family Physician* 76, no. 3 (2007): 391–96, http://www.aafp.org/afp/2007/0801/p391.html.

9. Eric Schoch, "Precision Prescribing," *The Art and Science of Medicine*, 2003, http://www.indiana.edu/~rcapub/v26n1/precision.shtml.

10. Martin Dawes, "The Implementation and Evaluation of Genetic Tests to Guide Drug Prescriptions in Primary Care in B.C.," in *What Is Personalized Medicine, and How Does It Affect You?* (Vancouver, BC, 2014). Public talk.

11. Colin J.D. Ross et al., "Genotypic Approaches to Therapy in Children: A National Active Surveillance Network (GATC) to Study the Pharmacogenomics of Severe Adverse Drug Reactions in Children," *Annals of the New York Academy of Sciences* 1110 (September 2007): 177–92.

12. Colin J.D. Ross et al., "Genetic Variants in TPMT and COMT Are Associated with Hearing Loss in Children Receiving Cisplatin Chemotherapy," *Nature Genetics* 45, no. 5 (April 26, 2013): 578.

13. Henk Visscher et al., "Pharmacogenomic Prediction of Anthracycline-Induced Cardiotoxicity in Children," *Journal of Clinical Oncology* 30, no. 13 (May 1, 2012): 1422–28.

14. J. Kirchheiner et al., "Pharmacokinetics of Codeine and Its Metabolite Morphine in Ultra-Rapid Metabolizers due to CYP2D6 Duplication," *The Pharmacogenomics Journal* 7, no. 4 (August 2007): 257–65.

15. G. Köhler and C. Milstein, "Continuous Cultures of Fused Cells Secreting Antibody of Predefined Specificity," *Nature* 256, no. 5517 (August 7, 1975): 495–97.

16. Mark D. Pegram, Gottfried Konecny, and Dennis J. Slamon, "The Molecular and Cellular Biology of HER2/neu Gene Amplification/ Overexpression and the Clinical Development of Herceptin (Trastuzumab) Therapy for Breast Cancer," in *Advances in Breast Cancer Management*, ed. William J. Gradishar and William C. Wood, vol. 103, Cancer Treatment and Research (Boston, MA: Springer, 2000), 57–75.

17. Richard Heimler, "Richard Heimler," *Lung Cancer Alliance*, accessed July 28, 2014, http://www.lungcanceralliance.org/get-help-and-support/ coping-with-lung-cancer/stories-of-hope/richard-heimler.html.

18. "FDA Approval for Crizotinib," *National Cancer Institute*, 2013, http://www.cancer.gov/cancertopics/druginfo/fda-crizotinib.

19. Kent Pinkerton, "Cystic Fibrosis Life Expectancy Statistics," *Disabled World*, 2009, http://www.disabled-world.com/health/respiratory/ cystic-fibrosis/ life-expectancy.php.

20. Bonnie W. Ramsey et al., "A CFTR Potentiator in Patients with Cystic Fibrosis and the G551D Mutation," *The New England Journal of Medicine* 365, no. 18 (November 3, 2011): 1663–72.

21. Alex Parker, "A Reflection...," *Kalydeco for Cystic Fibrosis Diary*, accessed July 28, 2014, http://kalydecoforaustralians.blogspot.ca/2012/11/ a-reflection.html.

22. Sining Chen and Giovanni Parmigiani, "Meta-Analysis of BRCA1 and BRCA2 Penetrance," *Journal of Clinical Oncology* 25, no. 11 (April 10, 2007): 1329–33.

23. Angelina Jolie, "My Medical Choice," *The New York Times*, May 14, 2013, http://www.nytimes.com/2013/05/14/opinion/my-medical -choice.html?_r=2&.

24. "SAP and BC Centre for Excellence in HIV/AIDS Pioneer New Technology, Redefine Treatment," *SAP News*, February 25, 2014, http://www.news-sap .com/sap-and-bc-centre-for-excellence-in-hiv-aids-pioneer-new-technology -redefine-treatment/.

25. Allen D. Roses, "On the Discovery of the Genetic Association of Apolipoprotein E Genotypes and Common Late-Onset Alzheimer Disease," *Journal of Alzheimer's Disease* 9, no. 3 Suppl (January 2006): 361–66, http://www.ncbi.nlm.nih.gov/pubmed/16914873.

26. Lindsay S. Nagamatsu et al., "Resistance Training Promotes Cognitive and Functional Brain Plasticity in Seniors with Probable Mild Cognitive Impairment," *Archives of Internal Medicine* 172, no. 8 (April 23, 2012): 666–68.

27. Elaine Westwick, "Huntington's Disease—Genetic Testing, Children and Hope," *The Stuff of Life*, July 2011, http://elainewestwick.blogspot.ca/2011/07/huntingtons -disease-genetic-testing.html.

28. Marilynn Marchione, "Texas Hospital Plans 'Moonshot' against Cancer," *AP: The Big Story*, 2012, http://bigstory.ap.org/article/texas-hospital-plans-moonshot-against-cancer.

29. Emily Dugan, "Thousands of NHS Patients to Have DNA Sequenced to Help Cancer Research," *The Independent*, July 20, 2014, http://www.independent.co.uk/life-style/health-and-families/health-news/thousands-of-nhs-patients-to-have-dna-sequenced-to -help-cancer-research-9617513.html.

30. Steven J.M. Jones et al., "Evolution of an Adenocarcinoma in Response to Selection by Targeted Kinase Inhibitors," *Genome Biology* 11, no. 8 (January 2010): R82.

31. Gina Kolata, "In Leukemia Treatment, Glimpses of the Future," *The New York Times*, July 8, 2012, http://www.nytimes.com/2012/07/08/health/in-gene-sequencing-treatment-for-leukemia-glimpses-of-the-future.html?pagewanted=all.

32. Xiao-jun Li et al., "A Blood-Based Proteomic Classifier for the Molecular Characterization of Pulmonary Nodules," *Science Translational Medicine* 5, no. 207 (October 16, 2013): 207ra142, doi:10.1126/scitranslmed.3007013.

33. Food and Drug Administration, "FDA Approves New Orphan Drug Kynamro to Treat Inherited Cholesterol Disorder," January 29, 2013, http://www.fda.gov/newsevents/newsroom/pressannouncements/ucm337195.htm.

34. Andrew Pollack, "Experimental Drug Used for Ebola-Related Virus Shows Promise," *The New York Times*, August 20, 2014, http://www.nytimes.com/2014/08/21/business/drug-used-for-ebola-related-virus-shows-promise.html?_r=0.

35. Giorgio Trinchieri, "Inflammation," in *Cancer: Principles and Practice of Oncology*, ed. Vincent T. DeVita Jr., Theodore S. Lawrence, and Steven A. Rosenberg, 9th ed. (Philadelphia: Lippincott Williams and Wilkins, 2011), http://www.lwwoncology.com/Textbook/Toc.aspx?id=11000#.

36. Penn Medicine, "Penn Medicine Team Reports Findings from Research Study of First 59 Adult and Pediatric Leukemia Patients Who Received Investigational, Personalized Cellular Therapy CTL019," December 7, 2013, http://www.uphs.upenn.edu/news/news_releases/2013/12/ctl019/.

37. Laura Smith-Spark, "UK Takes Step toward 'Three-Parent Babies,'" *CNN.com*, June 28, 2013, http://www.cnn.com/2013/06/28/health/ uk-health-dna-ivf/.

38. Dan Roden, "Engineering a Healthcare System to Deliver Personalized Medicine." Personalized Medicine and Individualized Drug Delivery, joint conference of the Canadian Society for Pharmaceutical Sciences and Canadian Chapter of Controlled Release Society, June 11–14, 2013, Vancouver.

39. *Association for Molecular Pathology et al. v. Myriad Genetics, Inc., et al.* 569 U.S. 12-398 (2013). http://www.supremecourt.gov/opinions/12pdf/ 12-398_1b7d.pdf.

40. Dan Munro, "FDA Slaps Personal Genomics Startup 23andMe with Stiff Warning," *Forbes*, November 25, 2013, http://www.forbes.com/ sites/danmunro/2013/11/25/fda-slaps-personal-genomics-startup -23andme-with-stiff-warning/.

41. Larry Husten, "Can Personalized Medicine and an Adaptive Trial Design Salvage This Hard-Luck Drug?," *Forbes*, December 4, 2013, http://www.forbes.com/sites/larryhusten/2013/12/04/can-personalized -medicine-and-an-adaptive-trial-design-salvage-this-hard-luck-drug/.

42. Elizabeth O Lillie et al., "The N-of-1 Clinical Trial: The Ultimate Strategy for Individualizing Medicine?," *Personalized Medicine* 8, no. 2 (March 2011): 161–73.

43. Jaime L Natoli et al., "Prenatal Diagnosis of Down Syndrome: A Systematic Review of Termination Rates (1995–2011)," *Prenatal Diagnosis* 32, no. 2 (February 2012): 142–53.

44. "Gendercide: The Worldwide War on Baby Girls," *The Economist*, March 4, 2010, http://www.economist.com/node/15636231.

CHAPTER 6

1. Salima Hacein-Bey-Abina et al., "Insertional Oncogenesis in 4 Patients after Retrovirus-Mediated Gene Therapy of SCID-X1," *The Journal of Clinical Investigation* 118, no. 9 (September 2, 2008): 3132–42.

2. Sheryl Gay Stolberg, "The Biotech Death of Jesse Gelsinger," *The New York Times*, November 28, 1999, http://www.nytimes.com/1999/11/28/ magazine/the-biotech-death-of-jesse-gelsinger.html.

3. Bill Clinton, "Remarks on the Completion of the First Survey of the Entire Human Genome Project" (The White House Office of the Press Secretary, 2000), http://clinton5.nara.gov/WH/New/html/ genome-20000626.html.

4. European Medicines Agency, "European Medicines Agency Recommends First Gene Therapy for Approval," July 20, 2012, http://www.ema.europa .eu/ema/index .Jsp?curl=pages/news_and_events/news/2012/07/ news_detail_001574.Jsp&mid =wc0b01ac058004d5c1.

5. Food and Drug Administration, "FDA Approves New Orphan Drug Kynamro to Treat Inherited Cholesterol Disorder," January 29, 2013, http://www.fda.gov/newsevents/newsroom/pressannouncements/ ucm337195.htm.

6. Alnylam Pharmaceuticals, "Alnylam Reports Positive Phase II Data for Patisiran (ALN-TTR02), an RNAi Therapeutic Targeting Transthyretin (TTR) for the Treatment of TTR-Mediated Amyloidosis (ATTR), and Initiates Phase III Trial," 2013, http://investors.alnylam.com/ releasedetail.cfm?ReleaseID=805999.

7. Aaron Krol, "Gene Therapy's Next Generation," *Bio-IT World*, January 29, 2014, http://www.bio-itworld.com/2014/1/29/gene-therapys-next -generation.html.

8. Mark J. Graham et al., "Antisense Inhibition of Proprotein Convertase Subtilisin/kexin Type 9 Reduces Serum LDL in Hyperlipidemic Mice," *Journal of Lipid Research* 48, no. 4 (April 1, 2007): 763–67.

9. María M Corrada et al., "Dementia Incidence Continues to Increase with Age in the Oldest Old: The 90+ Study," *Annals of Neurology* 67, no. 1 (January 2010): 114–21.

10. Michael D. Hurd et al., "Monetary Costs of Dementia in the United States," *New England Journal of Medicine* 368 (2013): 1326–34.

11. National Institute of Mental Health, "The Numbers Count: Mental Disorders in America," *National Institute of Mental Health*, accessed July 28, 2014, http://www.nimh.nih.gov/health/publications/the-numbers -count-mental-disorders-in-america/index.shtml.

12. Rafael Yuste and George M. Church, "The New Century of the Brain," *Scientific American* 310, no. 3 (February 18, 2014): 38–45.

13. Mark W. Stanton, *The High Concentration of U.S. Health Care Expenditures* (Washington, DC: U.S. Department of Health and Human Services, Public Health Services, Agency for Healthcare Research and Quality, 2006).

14. Canadian Institute for Health Information, *Seniors and the Health Care System: What Is the Impact of Multiple Chronic Conditions?*, 2011.

15. "Immortal Worms Defy Aging," *ScienceDaily*, February 27, 2012, http://www.sciencedaily.com/releases/2012/02/120227152612.htm.

16. Kathleen Y. Wolin and Hallie Tuchman, "Physical Activity and Gastrointestinal Cancer Prevention," in *Physical Activity and Cancer*, ed. Kerry S. Courneya and Christine Friedenreich, vol. 26 (Berlin: Springer Science and Business Media, 2010), 400; I.M. Lee and Y. Oguma, "Physical Activity," in *Cancer Epidemiology and Prevention*, ed. David Schottenfeld and Joseph F. Fraumeni, 3rd ed. (New York, NY: Oxford University Press, 2006), 1416; Kathy Matheson, "Exercising May Reduce Lung Cancer Risk," *The Washington Post*, December 12, 2006, http://www.washingtonpost.com/wp-dyn/content/article/2006/12/12/AR2006121200862.html; "Caffeine and Exercise May Be Protective against Skin Cancer Caused by Sun Exposure, Study Suggests," *ScienceDaily*, April 3, 2012, http://www.sciencedaily.com/releases/2012/04/120403142328.htm.

17. Paul D. Thompson et al., "Exercise and Physical Activity in the Prevention and Treatment of Atherosclerotic Cardiovascular Disease: A Statement from the Council on Clinical Cardiology (Subcommittee on Exercise, Rehabilitation, and Prevention) and the Council on Nutrition, Physical," *Circulation* 107, no. 24 (June 24, 2003): 3109–16.

18. Rob Stein, "Exercise Could Slow Aging of Body, Study Suggests," *The Washington Post*, January 29, 2008, http://www.washingtonpost.com/wp-dyn/content/article/2008/01/28/AR2008012801873.html.

19. Steve Horvath, "DNA Methylation Age of Human Tissues and Cell Types," *Genome Biology* 14, no. 10 (January 2013): R115.

20. Elaine Schmidt, "UCLA Scientist Uncovers Biological Clock Able to Measure Age of Most Human Tissues," *UCLA Newsroom*, October 21, 2013, http://newsroom.ucla.edu/releases/ucla-scientist-uncovers-biological-248950.

21. Manisha Sinha et al., "Restoring Systemic GDF11 Levels Reverses Age-Related Dysfunction in Mouse Skeletal Muscle," *Science* 344, no. 6184 (May 9, 2014): 649–52.

22. Robert Langreth, "Venter Starts DNA-Scanning Company to Boost Longevity," *Bloomberg.com*, March 4, 2014, http://www.bloomberg.com/news/2014-03-04/venter-starts-dna-scanning-company-to-boost-longevity.html; Saul A. Villeda et al., "Young Blood Reverses Age-Related Impairments in Cognitive Function and Synaptic Plasticity in Mice," *Nature Medicine* 20, no. 6 (June 2014): 659–63; Lida Katsimpardi et al., "Vascular and Neurogenic Rejuvenation of the Aging Mouse Brain by Young Systemic Factors," *Science* 344, no. 6184 (May 9, 2014): 630–34.

23. Jane Wakefield, "Google Spin-off Calico to Search for Answers to Ageing," *BBC News*, September 19, 2013, http://www.bbc.com/news/technology-24158924.

24. William J. Broad, "Billionaires with Big Ideas Are Privatizing American Science," *The New York Times*, March 16, 2014, http://www.nytimes.com/2014/03/16/science/billionaires-with-big-ideas-are-privatizing-american-science.html?_r=0.

25. L. Bellows, R. Moore, and A. Gross, "Dietary Supplements: Vitamins and Minerals" (University of Colorado Extension, 2013), http://www.ext.colostate.edu/pubs/foodnut/09338.html.

26. Leroy Hood and Nathan D. Price, "Promoting Wellness and Demystifying Disease: The 100K Project," *Genetic Engineering and Biotechnology News*, May 22, 2014.

27. "Biomarkers in Blood Show Potential as Early Detection Method of Pancreatic Cancer," *ScienceDaily*, January 21, 2014, http://www.sciencedaily.com/releases/2014/01/140121164754.htm.

28. "Detecting Dementia through microRNA in Patient Blood Samples," *Biome*, October 2, 2013, http://www.biomedcentral.com/biome/detecting-dementia-through-microrna-in-patient-blood-samples/.

29. John Ericson, "A Breath Test For Lung Cancer: Researchers Develop Biomarker for Pulmonary Tumor Growth," *Medical Daily*, October 18, 2013, http://www.medicaldaily.com/breath-test-lung-cancer-researchers-develop-biomarker-pulmonary-tumor-growth-261201.

30. "Intel Science Winner Develops Cancer Tech," *Wall Street Journal Live*, December 30, 2012, http://live.wsj.com/video/intel-science-winner-develops-cancer-tech/E342B43B-F184-492D-A441-38B28C18D3C1.HTML#!E342B43B-F184-492D-A441-38B28C18D3C1.

31. "Genomic Test Accurately Sorts Viral versus Bacterial Infections," *Duke University Pratt School of Engineering*, September 18, 2013, http://www.pratt.duke.edu/news/genomic-test-accurately-sorts-viral-versus-bacterial-infections.

32. Sarah C.P. Williams, "One Drug to Shrink All Tumors," *Science News*, March 26, 2012, http://news.sciencemag.org/health/2012/03/one-drug-shrink-all-tumors.

33. "Surprising Variation among Genomes of Individual Neurons from Same Brain," *ScienceDaily*, November 1, 2013, http://www.sciencedaily.com/releases/2013/11/131101172313.htm.

34. David J. Hill, "Patient Receives 3D Printed Implant to Replace 75 Percent of Skull," *Singularity Hub*, March 28, 2013, http://singularityhub.com/2013/03/28/patient-receives-3d-printed-implant-to-replace-75-percent-of-skull/.

35. Dan Howarth, "3D-Printed Eye Cells Could 'Cure Blindness,'" *Dezeen*, December 18, 2013, http://www.dezeen.com/2013/12/18/3d-printed-eye-cells-could-cure-blindness/.

36. "Use of Stem Cells in Personalized Medicine," *ScienceDaily*, November 26, 2012, http://www.sciencedaily.com/releases/2012/11/121126151021.htm.

37. Institute of Medicine (U.S.) Forum on Drug Discovery, Development, and Translation, "Introduction," in *Addressing the Barriers to Pediatric Drug Development: Workshop Summary* (Washington, DC: National Academies Press, 2008), http://www.ncbi.nlm.nih.gov/books/NBK3989/.

38. John Sloan, *A Bitter Pill: How The Medical System Is Failing The Elderly* (Vancouver, BC: Greystone Books, 2009), p. 29.

39. Paul Cerrato, "Why Personal Health Records Have Flopped," *InformationWeek*, January 12, 2012, http://www.informationweek.com/healthcare/patient-tools/why-personal-health-records-have-flopped/d/d-id/1102247?.

40. "An Update on Google Health and Google PowerMeter," *Official Google Blog*, June 24, 2011, http://googleblog.blogspot.ca/2011/06/update-on-google-health-and-google.html.

CHAPTER 7

1. Stanislaw Ulam, "Tribute to John von Neumann," *Bulletin of the American Mathematical Society* 64, no. 3 (1958): 5.

2. "Ray Kurzweil Biography," *Kurzweil Accelerating Intelligence*, accessed September 12, 2014, http://www.kurzweilai.net/ray-kurzweil-biography.

3. Ray Kurzweil, *The Singularity Is Near: When Humans Transcend Biology* (New York: Viking, 2005).

INDEX

CONQUERING
LYME DISEASE